The

Yates
Protocol

The
Yates
Protocol

Five Simple Steps to Fix Your Blood Sugar
and Reverse Type 2 Diabetes

Dr. Beverly Yates

AVERY
an imprint of Penguin Random House
New York

AVERY

an imprint of Penguin Random House LLC
1745 Broadway, New York, NY 10019
penguinrandomhouse.com

Most Avery books are available at a discount when purchased in quantity for sales promotions or corporate use. Special editions, which include personalized covers, excerpts, and corporate imprints, can be created when purchased in large quantities. For more information, please e-mail specialmarkets@penguinrandomhouse.com. Your local bookstore can also assist with discounted bulk purchases using the Penguin Random House corporate Business-to-Business program. For assistance in locating a participating retailer, e-mail B2B@penguinrandomhouse.com.

Book design by Angie Boutin

LIBRARY OF CONGRESS CATALOGING-IN-PUBLICATION DATA
Names: Yates, Beverly author
Title: The Yates protocol : five simple steps to fix your blood sugar and reverse type 2 diabetes / Dr. Beverly Yates.
Description: New York : Avery, an imprint of Penguin Random House, [2026] | Includes bibliographical references and index.
Identifiers: LCCN 2025025630 (print) | LCCN 2025025631 (ebook) |
ISBN 9780593852996 hardcover | ISBN 9780593853009 ebook
Subjects: LCSH: Diabetes—Diet therapy—Popular works | Blood glucose monitoring—Popular works
Classification: LCC RC660.4 .Y38 2026 (print) | LCC RC660.4 (ebook)
LC record available at https://lccn.loc.gov/2025025630
LC ebook record available at https://lccn.loc.gov/2025025631

Printed in the United States of America
1st Printing

The authorized representative in the EU for product safety and compliance is Penguin Random House Ireland, Morrison Chambers, 32 Nassau Street, Dublin D02 YH68, Ireland, https://eu-contact.penguin.ie.

This book is dedicated to those who want a clear, sustainable path forward. May you find inspiration, clarity, and practical steps on this healing journey.

CONTENTS

I
The Five Steps

· · · · · · · · · · · · · · ·

II
Implementation

· · · · · · · · · · · · · ·

III
Deeper Dives

· · · · · · · · · · · · · ·

Prologue

You're fat, you're lazy, it's your own damn fault!

Maria got in the car and threw the stack of pamphlets on the passenger seat, slamming the door shut behind her.

She gripped the steering wheel tight and leaned forward to rest her head on her hands. She took a few big, heaving breaths, trying not to cry—not over this, not again.

She had just left the doctor's office. It was the twelfth doctor she'd seen in three years.

"Just focus on reducing food intake," he'd gently suggested to her.

"I don't eat badly!" she'd said quickly. "Normally, I eat really well, low sugar with lots of salads! I've been trying a keto diet recently . . ." As usual, it felt like he wasn't listening to what she had to say.

"And, here, take a look at these."

He'd thrust a stack of pamphlets at her. She already knew what they'd be about: Ozempic, Mounjaro, Wegovy, Jardiance, etc. All classic type 2 drugs. And of course, Metformin as the basic starter medication. After twelve doctors pushing the same pre-scriptions, she knew these brochures by heart.

But as she kept trying to tell them, *prescriptions weren't what she wanted. The side effects and risks scared her. Was she going to be stuck on them for life? Would they remain effective? Or would she walk the tightrope of high risk for heart disease, strokes, vision loss, kidney disease, dialysis, amputation, and other complications from diabetes and blood sugar problems, for the rest of her life? Would she lose her independence and need her kids to take care of her?*

Maria was at a loss. What could she do? She knew *type 2 was reversible . . . She was trying* so hard. *She worked out! She dieted! But doctors often took one look at her diagnosis, one look at her chart, and one look at her belly. She sometimes saw it in their eyes, just like in some of her friends and colleagues:* Just stop being so lazy. *She wasn't lazy! She wasn't choosing to have diabetes!*

Why was she constantly shamed and blamed for having this disease, even though she was putting so much time and effort into fighting it? Maria didn't choose to make herself sick. But it was getting that much harder each time to ask for help, again.

Maria sighed. She felt her hope slipping. Where was the care, the help, the authenticity, the humanity *in all this? Was she doomed to struggle alone?*

Introduction

My name is Dr. Beverly Yates. I'm genetically vulnerable to type 2 and prediabetes—and highly aware of what it takes to reverse type 2 and prevent it in the first place.

My father was one of thirteen siblings who each had some type of diabetes. Each suffered from terrible complications, and each died before their time.

I didn't start out as a doctor. I went to MIT in the '80s and graduated with a bachelor of science degree in electrical engineering. I started out working as a systems engineer in Silicon Valley in my early twenties. When we moved to the Silicon Forest area of metro Portland, Oregon, I suddenly became very ill. Doctors couldn't figure out what was wrong. Was I doomed? Was I going to keep getting worse? I was terrified. Initially, I saw no way out. But then I had one of the most important realizations of my life: The body is a biological *system*. I was a systems specialist. Could I use my training in analyzing complex systems to figure out what was causing my issues and heal myself?

As it turns out, I could. I found the underlying cause of my symptoms, addressed it, and got better. And that experience made me wonder: Could I do the same for other people?

DIABETES IS COMPLICATED

Diabetes is complicated. If I have learned one thing in all my work with diabetic and prediabetic patients, it's that it is a complex phenomenon. **Every person's experience is unique.** My father's side of the family is evidence of this: symptoms, blood sugar levels, reactions to foods that spike blood sugar, what makes things better or worse—it's all so different, even within families. In my clinic I've seen twins have totally different blood sugar experiences. A "one size fits all" approach makes things worse, not better. There is an apt saying: *If you've seen one person with type 2 diabetes, you've seen one person with type 2 diabetes.* You can make no assumptions about anybody else! Type 2 and prediabetes are complex.

Our society, often including health professionals, treats type 2 diabetes and other blood sugar issues like they are easy to fix. It's a sad but true reality: Humans instinctively oversimplify and judge. In our culture, there's an overlap between people who have high body fat percentages and people who have type 2 and prediabetes. So, the basic conclusion most people leap to is:

Body fat is the cause of type 2 and prediabetes. You have type 2 or prediabetes because you're too lazy to eat right and exercise.

I left Silicon Valley, went to naturopathic medical school and began practicing naturopathic medicine in the mid-90s. My work in systems engineering enabled me to see instantly the absurdity of this oversimplified conclusion—and all the shame and blame that result. I saw right away that not only were health professionals and researchers leaping to preemptive conclusions, but there was something deeply wrong with the science. It was missing crucial details and nuance.

For example, poor sleep and stress are two major causes of type 2 and prediabetes. They have been overlooked for decades. Up until a few years ago, almost no major studies probed the roles of sleep and stress in type 2 and prediabetes.

Meanwhile, I saw major blood sugar effects of both sleep and stress instantly in my clinical practice. It's clear when you work one on one with people and get to know them as whole beings.

PATIENT EXPERIENCES SHOW WHAT WORKS

In the mid-2000s, I noticed a steep rise in people coming into my clinic with type 2 and prediabetes. Most of them came to me saying the same thing: *I'm trying so hard; I'm not getting better.* Some had been seeing doctor after doctor, often dragged by their adult children or other family members, without finding any real help or support. Almost everybody was coming to me discouraged. Shamed. Frustrated. Afraid. Losing hope.

I was also learning about the extent of devastation that diabetes had wrought on my own family. My parents divorced when I was one year old, and I didn't grow up with my biological father's side of the family in my life as a child. When I gathered my courage as an adult and established a relationship with my father, I discovered what a wrecking ball diabetes was in this side of the family. I was unaware of my increased risks for diabetes until I got to know this side of my genetic family. What an important reveal this was!

I committed myself to developing a deeper understanding of type 2 and prediabetes. I committed myself to figuring out how to *reverse type 2*, for *good*—something many people know is possible but none of the conventional approaches were even close to doing.

I tapped the most important—and almost entirely ignored—source of information on type 2 and prediabetes there are:

Patient experiences.

I asked questions like:

What genes were my patients born with? Were they breastfed? What kinds of environments were they raised in? Have they been on antibiotics? Have they gone through major traumas? Have they been exposed to environmental toxins? Do they have major food sensitivities? Are they stressed? Do they sleep long and deep? Do they have access to healthy foods?

Together, we found answers. We found small, sustainable changes that restored their damaged metabolisms. Such tweaks included adding leafy greens to breakfast, going on a walk after dinner, or installing blackout drapes in their bedrooms.

Contrary to all the shame, blame, and one-size-fits-all answers that dominate traditional approaches, patient experiences proved to me beyond a shadow of a doubt that the causes of type 2 and prediabetes are not anyone's fault—*and* that the way to heal them isn't willpower or restriction. Change is never easy, but it doesn't require superhuman efforts.

The answer is simple: *heal.*

Heal. Type 2 and prediabetes come from damage to your metabolism, specifically what I refer to throughout this book as your metabolic machinery, because there are many organs and systems that need to be in good health for metabolism—including managing blood sugar—to work. Healing doesn't happen when you force yourself into dieting and exercise extremes. Healing happens when you restore nutrient status, reduce inflammation, regain harmony and balance with your body, bit by bit.

Healing happens with feasible, sustainable tweaks to daily habits. Healing happens when you get on your body's side, nourish it, and improve the health of your metabolism one day at a time.

That's *it.*

DAMAGE AND OVERLOOKED CAUSES

Type 2 and prediabetes occur when the body's blood sugar management system—that metabolic machinery—gets *damaged.* Body fat, especially visceral abdominal fat around the organs, and a sedentary lifestyle can play a role in this. But those are just two of so many causes of damage, which include excessive antibiotic use, environmental toxins, chronic or severe stress, childhood trauma, viral illnesses, and poor sleep. These causes can plant seeds of damage that then ping-pong around in the body and progressively worsen under the radar for *decades*. **Type 2 and prediabetes aren't conditions of willpower. They are conditions of *damage*.**

I have had clients whose diet and exercise habits were perfect in every respect: They got type 2 or prediabetes anyway! Sometimes people's kitchens are brimming over with healthy foods. Genes play a role in how vulnerable any of us are; one of my patients, Joseph, is a male in his twenties with excellent diet and fitness, tons of muscle, and basically no body fat, but he's got a lot of genetic markers that make him more vulnerable to blood sugar dysregulation. Other factors are always in play.

Another patient, Sandra, pushed over from prediabetes to type 2 when she started working nights. Sandra became diabetic after taking on extra responsibilities at work and starting to sleep just five hours a night. I've had perfectly healthy patients become prediabetic after weathering major disturbances to their gut microbiomes. Corey recently became prediabetic after contracting Lyme disease while going through a stressful divorce.

Poor sleep and stress cause inflammation and oxidative stress, damaging the metabolic machinery. They disrupt key hormones that regulate appetite, making it impossible to tell when you're full.

Type 2 diabetes is multicausal, and always arises due to damage. It is healed by healing damage.

THE SOLUTION ISN'T DISCIPLINE

I've worked with thousands of people on their blood sugar over the course of thirty years. There is only *one* trait I've found they all share:

None of them chose to have type 2 or prediabetes or blood sugar dysregulation out of laziness.

In fact, many of my patients are the most hardworking and self-sacrificing people I've met. In this book you'll meet Len, a retiree who spent thirty-one years in the military and now volunteers to support other veterans,

Sonia, who cares for an adult child with a seizure disorder,

Janalee, a successful entrepreneur and business owner,

Sandra, who works two jobs, sleeps five hours a night, and burns the candle at both ends to support her family,

Reverend Lorraine, pastor to a congregation of three hundred,

Dina and Edna, both committed to healing themselves so their children aren't forced to become their caregivers as they age,

Joanna, a nurse who works eighteen-hour shifts and who has always been so sacrificial with her family that when she told them she had type 2 diabetes, they literally couldn't believe it: *But you're the one who's supposed to care for us,* they said.

These people are the norm, not the exception.

It's said that people with diabetes don't work hard enough, but the truth, if anything, is usually the opposite: They're working too hard! I see patterns: veterans, shift workers, emergency service workers, hospital employees, caretakers, first responders. People working two jobs. People who care for ill family members. People taking care of children and their aging parents at the same time. People getting divorced.

And the disease is absolutely exhausting. It drags your organs through the mud, slams your blood sugar up and down, disrupts sleep, causes weight gain, and taxes your already struggling digestive, immune, and nervous systems. And yet? You and everyone else are at the mercy of it and told to *keep going.*

I know whatever your circumstances are, you didn't choose them. I'm here for you with insight from experience. Providing information you can use to build new habits that heal you and set you free from the risks of blood sugar danger.

THE FIVE STEPS OF HEALTH: NUTRITION, MEAL TIMING, SLEEP, EXERCISE & STRENGTH TRAINING, AND STRESS

I've identified five major domains of health where making improvements heals the underlying damage causing type 2 and prediabetes:

Nutrition, meal timing, exercise & strength training, sleep, and stress.

All five steps are important elements of overall health. Yet in my clinic, people succeed even when they implement one step at a time and focus on two, and no more than three, steps overall. Many people can or need to make changes across the board, but almost all are best served by starting with one and building from there.

I invite you to first learn about all five steps, then identify which could help you most. Choose *one* of these to implement first.

Most influencers recommend extreme diets: very low carb, or very low fat, or very low calorie, or vegan. While these plans might offer short-term blood sugar reprieve, they are usually disasters for long-term health. Extreme changes for short periods of time almost always make people *worse*.

I take the psychology of change very seriously. **The key to long-term health is building sustainable habits.** Focus on what is most feasible and likely to help you at this moment. Once it becomes habituated and second nature, add more. All along, you're healing yourself so you're gaining energy and the capacity to do more.

When I first met Maria, she was making every mistake in the book. She was stressed, had a poor diet, no proper meal timing or rhythm, no real exercise or movement, terrible sleep interrupted by searing heartburn from her heavy late dinners. She needed help with everything.

But we started with one step: meal timing. A new meal schedule helped her appetite, cravings, and energy.

THE GOAL AND EXPECTATIONS

The goal is to bring your blood sugar numbers down. Your progress doesn't have to be perfectly linear, but the trend is down. Back into healthier ranges: down from diabetes into prediabetes (remission), then down into full reversal.

When you start the Yates Protocol, you should see noticeable improvement within a few weeks. Depending on the extent of the changes you make, it could even be sooner.

There is one major indicator of blood sugar health that many people know to focus on: hemoglobin A1C, which is a measure of average blood sugar over the past three months. If you have type 2, the first big goal is "remission," which is getting the A1C down from above the diabetic level of 6.5 percent to below 6.5. This is a win. But you can keep going. When you bring your A1C down to 5.6 percent or lower, that's "reversal." Ideally, you get it even lower, between 4.8 and 5.4 percent. It's certainly possible. Many people can get down into this completely reversed state. Some people can get close. It's context dependent. Celebrate your wins, keep dialing in.

Reversal isn't "cure." Once you begin implementing the Yates Protocol, you must keep doing it. That's why it's so important to do it sustainably and enjoyably.

GETTING STARTED

It's remarkable to me how quickly people's bodies can respond to even the smallest of changes, the tiniest first steps on this path. No matter what your situation is right now, you have an amazing opportunity for healing. I also know change is never easy, but it is easier together. I'm here with you and for you. Let's make progress and keep it going.

I

The Five Steps

CHAPTER 1

Nutrition

Eat Smarter, Not Harder, with These
4 Blood-Sugar-Friendly Food Groups

CHAPTER MAP

. . . .

This chapter explains what to eat and why.

KEY SECTIONS

. . . .

- The four food groups of the Yates Protocol
- Hydration
- Successful foraging: how to identify and buy healthful foods
- Nutrition labels: how to avoid being tricked

Stan walked into my office and greeted me with a direct smile and firm handshake. Like many of my patients, his face had some lines of worry and discouragement carved in it after repeated difficulty with conventional health care. But he arrived for his first appointment optimistic and eager to improve his health.

Stan's A1C was 10 percent. I wanted to start bringing it down ASAP. I thought nutrition was the place to start. He said he was eating mostly premade meals from the freezer section of the grocery store. I told him this isn't necessarily the worst thing in the world, but it is often detrimental. I asked: "Which meals? Can you show me the packaging?"

The meals were savory, but they often contained pasta and white rice, which are simple sugars that spike blood sugar, unhealthy fats and additives, and sweetened sauces and dressings.

I told Stan he would benefit immediately from changing what he was eating.

He sighed.

He explained: He just didn't want to learn to cook. It's not that he felt incapable or unmotivated, but his wife used to do all the cooking, and she had recently passed away. He said: "It's just not something I want to do right now."

"Okay," I said. "There's a way for you. Let's find it."

I gave Stan a simple plan: Focus on protein and leafy greens. Eat those first. Fill the rest of your plate with healthy fats and complex carbs/resistant starches. That was all Stan needed to start seeing improvement.

"Make this your home base, Stan. Always choose from what's available to you in those four groups." Stan was a veteran and invited to all sorts of luncheons. He agreed to be wary of gravy, dressings, sauces, and fried foods. He agreed to fill his plate with lean, unbreaded protein and vegetables first.

Then we talked about cooking. It turned out Stan's kids came by in the evenings and sometimes prepared meals for him. He spoke with his kids about his needs, and we invited his daughter to one of my online programs. Getting the kids more involved was a win for everybody.

Stan began seeing improvement in his post-meal blood sugar numbers, from about 100 mg/dl down to 50 mg/dl, and then with some more time down to 30–40 mg/dl, just where I like to see it. Soon after, his A1C decreased and he reached remission.

Nutrition is the bull's-eye at the center of health. Everything you eat is either incorporated into your body or excreted as waste. Those are the only two options.

When you eat something ultra-processed, highly refined, nutrient-poor, inflammatory, or otherwise destructive, it enters your body and has negative effects. It's like building a house out of something like sticks, which are the wrong materials. Ultra-processed foods are bad building materials and make the body more vulnerable to stress than houses made of bricks. End of story.

When you eat nourishing, vitamin-rich, nutrient-dense, anti-inflammatory foods, you give your body great building materials. You support the healthy organ and system function you were designed for. Healthy omega 3 fats from a fillet of salmon get folded into the structure of your brain. The calcium from broccoli becomes a part of your thigh bone. Tryptophan from a slice of turkey becomes a part of melatonin, the hormone your brain uses to put you to sleep. You're building the house of your body out of bricks!

To do this, you don't have to go on any extreme diets or even necessarily give up your favorite foods. You don't have to give up carbs, or fat, or meat, or go super low-calorie—not any of that diet culture mess.

In this chapter, I explain four categories of food—fiber, lean protein, healthy fat, and complex carbs/resistant starches.

THE FOUR FOOD GROUPS OF THE YATES PROTOCOL

Dieticians usually break down food into three major categories called *macronutrients*: fat, protein, and carbohydrates. *Macro* means *big*. They're the three big categories of food.

I have added a fourth: fiber. Fiber, while technically a carbohydrate, is indigestible to humans. It's a part of plants. It's the rough stuff like shells, skin, peels, seeds, and bark. This makes it very different from other carbohydrates—different enough, I think, that it should be considered a separate group.

Our culture abides by some major myths about macronutrients and type 2 and prediabetes. Some people think you need to eat a super low-carbohydrate diet. Others think you need to eat low fat. Such trends are always coming and going.

The truth is each macronutrient contains foods that can nourish you and play an important role in health. Yes, there are unhealthy carbs, and there are unhealthy fats. They harm health, *big-time*. But there are *healthy* carbs and fats that nourish you, too.

THE TEMPLATE FOR BUILDING A MEAL

On the Yates Protocol, fill every plate with the four groups.

The ideal breakdown:

- 50 percent of your plate is high-fiber vegetables, with a focus on leafy greens.

- 25 percent is lean protein.

- 25 percent is complex carbohydrate/resistant starch.

Fat is what you cook with or drizzle on top. It's cooking oil, dressings, and sauces. It is also often a part of lean proteins, as it's a natural (and healthy) component of meat, fish, and eggs.

FIBER

Start building your plate with high-fiber vegetables, with a focus on leafy greens. Fiber is the foundation of every blood-sugar-friendly meal.

Fiber is a part of plants, the rough stuff the human gut doesn't digest. The "meat" of any fruit, vegetable, or squash is naturally fibrous, but the most fibrous part is the skin: Think of apple, peach, or potato skin.

Fiber is what makes the difference between white rice products and the rest. Brown rice and other whole rice varieties have fiber because they have the bran—the little brown, black, red, or purple shell—on them. White rice has no fiber because the bran has been taken off. Most don't think of white rice as a processed food, but it is.

The same goes for wheat products: Whole grain products are fibrous because they still have the bran on them. Processed, refined (often called white) grain products do not. I call the bran of wheat and rice products a "fiber jacket." It's important to understand that while whole grain and rice products are often advertised as "high in fiber," that's only relative to their processed cousins. They have *much* less fiber than fruits and vegetables. They are *not* a part of the *fiber* food group.

Fiber is a blood-sugar sponge. Blood sugar (aka glucose) gets into your blood by being absorbed through your intestinal walls. When in your gut all on its own, blood sugar zips through the gut lining and puts you on a blood-sugar roller coaster, rocketing up and then crashing back down. But fiber takes up room in the gut and slows the absorption, preventing both spikes and crashes. It keeps you balanced, off the blood-sugar roller coaster.

Fiber promotes health for other reasons, too. It:

- is rich and healthy food for gut bacteria and directly feeds your microbiome;

- helps reduce intestinal permeability, therefore protecting you from toxins that enter the bloodstream and cause inflammation;

- improves cholesterol profiles. Fiber helps prevent the blood from getting sticky, so lowers the risks of inappropriate blood clotting, strokes, and heart attacks, lowers inflammation, boosts levels of the healthy HDL cholesterol, and decreases the amounts of triglycerides and unhealthy LDL;

- helps make it easier to tell when you are full. It takes up room in the gut, creating fullness, and helps you feel satisfied after eating meals so you know when to stop eating; and

- helps keep bowel movements regular.

Beans, peas, other legumes, nuts, and seeds are all naturally high in fiber. Berries are quite high in fiber: It's their rough skin, hair, and little seeds. They also tend to be lower in carbohydrates than other fruits.

The vegetables that are most likely to elevate blood sugar are the sweetest ones: corn (sometimes considered a grain), butternut squash, sweet potatoes, yams, and even carrots, tomatoes, and bell peppers. All fruits are likely to solicit a response, with berries potentially the lowest due to their high fiber content.

For all vegetables, focus on eating them in their most natural form: minimal processing, and skin on. For example, you can consume corn in so many different forms: creamed, in a can, frozen corn you cook at home, or fresh corn right off the cob. If you eat it off the cob and get all the fibrous husk with it, that's good, it counts as a vegetable. But if you eat it from a can or bag, it's lost some of its fiber. If you eat it in a premade meal like canned soup, it may have toxic oils and additives.

There is one source of fiber that stands out above the rest. It's the one you want to try to include in nearly all your meals: leafy greens.

Leafy greens include collard greens, kale, broccoli, chard, spinach, salad greens, arugula, bok choy, and more.

Leafy greens are not just super high in fiber but also high in nutrients and low in carbohydrates. They slow down the blood sugar response, help with appetite, improve insulin sensitivity, restore nutrients, and help heal the gut microbiome. Many of my patients find that just adding leafy greens or swapping out simple carbs for greens is an excellent way to get started with the Yates Protocol.

You can increase the amount of fiber in a meal by incorporating other fiber-rich plant foods. Nuts, seeds, beans, peas, other legumes, or fruits all add fiber to a meal. But they are additions. Always make sure 50 percent of your meal is fibrous vegetables.

PRO TIP: ADD HEALTHY FAT

Add some healthy fat like an olive oil dressing to leafy greens or other vegetables. Fat further slows the absorption of sugar into the gut. Plus, fat helps your body absorb what are called *fat soluble nutrients*. All nutrients are either fat- or water-soluble. Vitamins such as A, D, E, and K are *fat soluble*: You absorb them best when there is fat with them in the gut.

PRO TIP: JUST TRY THE GREENS!, LIKE ANNA

One of my patients, Anna, was a picky eater and did not like leafy greens when we met.

She quickly found many Yates Protocol foods she loved to eat, but she was still reticent about trying leafy greens. After a few weeks, she was continuing to experience post-meal blood sugar rises of around 50 mg/dl. I prefer to see it at 20–40 mg/dl. I suggested she try consuming one cup of leafy greens before dinner every day for one week. I also told her it can take some time for the taste buds to adjust to certain healthy foods if your taste buds have been hijacked and have adjusted to ultra-processed foods.

Anna did as I invited. The next time we met via telehealth, she was delighted. The leafy greens helped bring her blood sugar responses down, and she also felt more full and energized after meals.

She approached the greens like medicine at first. "I just chewed and swallowed!" But then she began to really enjoy them. She now loves my collard greens recipe (204). She makes it when meal prepping on the weekends and eats the dish every day.

"I never believed I'd enjoy greens. I'd have kept chewing and swallowing them like medicine if I'd had to. I feel so much better when I eat them. But I can't believe it, *my taste buds have a new love!*" she said, laughing.

LEAN PROTEIN

There's usually some kind of cultural war happening between carbs and fat, but most agree: Protein is essential.

Lean protein (with fiber) is the foundation of every blood-sugar-friendly meal. Lean protein and fiber are a power couple.

Lean protein is essential for most of the work in the body: It's the building block of organs, makes and repairs cells, catalyzes reactions, and facilitates the burning of energy. Without sufficient protein, you can lose immune system function, bone density, muscle mass, strength, mental clarity, mental health, and metabolic function. In general, people who eat sufficient protein have the most satiation after meals and fastest-burning metabolisms. Protein makes it easier to notice you are no longer hungry or you are full and therefore feel satisfied after eating a meal.

Everybody's protein needs are different, but a nice guideline is one palm-size portion of lean animal protein or a cup of plant protein per meal. If you don't have kidney disease, you can eat additional servings of protein daily, especially if you are looking to increase your muscle mass when doing strength training.

Protein is crucial for everybody, no matter your age. Many people eat less protein as they age, but this is a mistake. It's the opposite of what you should do. The older you get, the more important it is to keep your protein intake sufficient. This helps you maintain muscle, bone, and tissue strength.

There are both plant and animal sources of protein.

For animal protein, eggs, chicken, turkey, fish, seafood, and shellfish are great.

Beef, lamb, venison, buffalo, and pork are also great sources, if you get lean cuts—*no bacon or pork belly!*

Why "lean" cuts?

First, if you eat only fatty cuts of meat, like bacon, pork belly, and sausages, you get less protein.

Second, toxins are stored in fat. So, if you eat conventional, industrially raised meat products, you can end up with less healthy and more toxic meat.

Third, some people with type 2 or prediabetes are sensitive to high amounts of fat in the diet, especially saturated fat. It's best to err on the side of caution. You want to prioritize getting sufficient protein and avoid overwhelming your body with a ton of saturated fat.

Quality matters for animal protein. "Grass fed," "grass finished," "pasture raised," "wild caught" are usually more expensive than "normal" meats, but I invite you to think deeply about what we consider "normal" today: inhumane slaughterhouses where animals are fed the cheapest, most industrial slop on the market.

Grass-fed cows, lambs, and pigs, pasture-raised chicken and eggs, and wild-caught fish have healthier kinds of fat in them, fewer toxins, and more vitamins and nutrients than factory-farmed products.

This is an important area to spend the extra money. Your grocery bill could end up lower because you need less food.

Is saturated fat okay to eat as a part of your "lean protein"? The saturated fat in egg yolks and other animal products, *especially when grass-fed or pasture-raised*, is often a rich source of vitamins and nutrients. As an example, the yolk of an egg contains choline, a necessary nutrient for liver health and preventing fatty liver, a key driver of insulin resistance, prediabetes, and type 2. Egg yolks also contain cholesterol and lecithin. Both are important building blocks used by the body. Cholesterol is the substrate for sex hormones like estrogen, progesterone, and testosterone. Lecithin is important for a healthy gut, liver, brain, and other health benefits.

For a long time, scientists thought that eating cholesterol caused high cholesterol and heart disease, but it doesn't. We now know the truth: The body produces far more cholesterol than you eat. The body makes cholesterol when inflamed. It uses cholesterol to try to heal itself. So high LDL cholesterol and a poor cholesterol profile is a sign there's something wrong for sure . . . but not because there's saturated fat in your diet.

It may be especially important to include whole eggs in your diet—both the whites and the yolks. The whites contain protein. The yolk is all fat. The yolks are where all the vitamins and nutrients are, so don't toss them. Particularly important is a nutrient called *choline*. Choline is necessary for keeping the liver from becoming "fatty." A fatty liver is one of the key drivers of insulin resistance, prediabetes, and type 2. Look for pasture-raised eggs, or better yet, those sold from a local farm. You can test their nutrient level by the color of the yolk. The more golden, the more nutrient-dense!

PRO TIP: TRY ORGAN MEATS

Organ meats like liver, kidney, and heart are *packed* with nutrients—more so than muscle meats! They are lean. They are often the cheapest parts of the animal. This is a lot of bang for the buck. They are sustainable, too: Most people don't want to eat them, so they're usually just thrown away. If you don't like the taste, try cooking organs in coconut oil, using a lot of spices, stirring them into stir-fries, chilis, or soups, or grinding them into sausages. To get their nutrients, you can also buy spices made from organ meats.

Not a meat eater? There are plenty of quality sources of plant protein.

All beans, peas, other legumes, and nuts and seeds contain protein. They are never *just* protein, however: They are a mix of protein and complex carbohydrates (with a little bit of fat and fiber mixed in). A cup of black beans contains 15 grams of protein (the same as two large eggs). That's less than a palm-size portion of meat, which is around 25–30 grams, but comparable.

Nuts and seeds contain some protein, too, though they are mostly fat. They should usually be considered in the "healthy fats" bucket, but can add some protein to a meal in a pinch. The highest protein nuts are peanuts, almonds, and pistachios, which contain about 6–7 grams of protein per medium-size handful (1 ounce). The rest is fat, and a lot of it. This isn't a bad thing; it just means they are very filling.

If you are vegetarian, vegan, pescatarian, flexitarian, whole foods plant-based, or on a low-meat diet, you need to be careful to get enough protein and to make sure it's complete protein. I describe protein and other needs on plant-based diets in the Resources section on my website.

PRO TIP: EAT PROTEIN FIRST

Timing matters for blood sugar. Eat protein first. Fiber is a good second food group because it's a blood sugar sponge and helps expand the stomach, signaling fullness. If you're vegetarian or plant-based, you can follow this advice but pay attention to your blood sugar and experiment with what may work best for you, as plant protein contains carbohydrates. Your continuous glucose monitor can give you this precious data (see chapter 7).

SWAP THIS FOR THAT

Roasted nuts	→	Raw nuts seasoned at home
Egg whites	→	Whole eggs
Pork belly or bacon	→	Turkey bacon
Ground beef	→	Lean ground beef, grass-fed
Yogurt, cheese, cottage cheese	→	Chia seed, almond, or coconut yogurt
Breakfast cereal or bagel	→	Eggs, any way you like them
Rice or other grain	→	Beans, lentils, or another legume
Wheat pasta	→	Zucchini noodles

HEALTHY FATS

Fat is important for many reasons. Your brain is made of fat, your skin is made of fat, and your organs are protected by fat. Many vitamins (A, D, E, and K) are fat-soluble, meaning you need to eat fat to absorb them. Fat also stimulates your production of satiation hormones, playing a key role in helping you feel full and know when to stop eating.

But there are some bad fats you need to avoid.

The most important to avoid are *trans fats*. There are trace amounts of natural trans fats in animal products, but these are healthy. It's the trans fats made in laboratories that are dangerous. They are highly inflammatory and directly contribute to poor heart health and insulin resistance. If you avoid processed foods and cook at home, you should be in the clear. If you purchase processed food, read the label. There is an area on each nutrition label for *trans fat*, but if a trans fat is 0.4 gram or less per serving, the amount rounds down and it doesn't have to be listed there. To spot a trans fat on a nutrition label, read the *ingredient list*. Trans fats hide on nutrition labels as shortening, margarine, or hydrogenated or partially hydrogenated oil.

Second, avoid processed vegetable and seed oils, including vegetable, soybean, corn, safflower, and canola (rapeseed) oil. They're in almost all processed foods because they are inexpensive, have a long shelf life, and have little flavor. They are also almost always used as the cooking oil or in dressings at restaurants, so be wary when dining out, too.

One tablespoon of these oils is the equivalent of many dozens, or even hundreds, of the seeds in them. This is an unnaturally high quantity to consume. Plus, the primary kind of fat in these products is omega 6 polyunsaturated fatty acid. Omega 6 is essential, but in small amounts. There is so much omega 6 in processed foods that it has been estimated that Americans consume more than fifteen times the necessary amount, contributing to inflammation, excess pain, dysregulated immune function, impaired heart health, and damage to metabolic machinery. Plus, these fats have often been processed at high temperatures, which oxidizes them, rendering them toxic to human tissues. They have had most of the nutrients stripped along the way, and unnatural chemicals are often used in the refining process. These can be very toxic.

A final important fat to avoid is deep-fried food—100 percent of the time. Commit to it. The oil used for deep-frying is usually processed seed oil. That's already a red flag. But deep-frying makes it worse: It reheats these already highly unstable oils repeatedly to the highest temperatures possible. This creates an extraordinary amount of inflammation and toxic by-products. The good news is there are easy swaps for heathier versions of your favorite fried foods. Check out my delicious recipe for Unfried Chicken on page 205.

Fortunately, many healthy fats remain.

First are the fats from lean protein: fat from grass-fed beef, lamb, pork, pasture-raised poultry and eggs.

There's also the fat of fatty fish and seafood. I didn't discuss this under "lean protein" because these fats—omega 3s—are special and deserve special attention. Omega 3s are the anti-inflammatory complement to the inflammatory omega 6s. Fatty fish rich in omega 3s include salmon, tuna, trout, anchovies, sardines, herring, and mackerel. Their skin and eggs (called *roe* or *caviar*) are also very high in omega 3s. I recommend 3–4 servings of fatty fish a week. Focus on wild-caught fish, since they usually have more nutrients in them and lower levels of potential contaminants like mercury (beware of tuna for possible mercury contamination—light and skipjack tuna have lower levels of mercury).

Butter is a saturated fat (it's about 99 percent fat, with some trace milk protein in it) rich in fat-soluble vitamins A, D, E, and K. Grass-fed butter is worth the few extra dollars: It's much higher in nutrients, including a precious molecule called *butyrate* that protects the gut lining from perforation and supports healthy appetite signaling. Just as with egg yolks, you can tell the nutrient density from looking at the color: brighter and deeper, like a darker gold or even orange color, means more nutrients.

I typically advise against consuming dairy for most people, but butter and ghee are the exception. The potentially problematic parts of dairy are the carbohydrate (lactose) and protein (casein and whey) due to the difficulty many people have in digesting it after early childhood. Since butter is 99 percent fat, you sidestep those issues. If you are very sensitive to the protein's casein or whey, try **ghee**, which is butter that has been boiled and stripped of even the trace amounts of these proteins, leaving only the fat and the vitamins behind.

Avocados are composed mostly of a rare, heart-healthy kind of fat called monounsaturated fat. Raw avocado and extra-virgin, cold-pressed avocado oil are excellent parts of a healthy diet.

Olives and olive oil are also rich sources of the precious monounsaturated fats.

But be wary: Cheap, oxidized (aka rancid) olive oil is everywhere. This is another place where it's worth it to spend a bit more money for higher quality.

Heat and light cause all unsaturated fats, mostly polyunsaturated fats but also these heart-healthy monounsaturated fats, to *oxidize*. Oxidized fats are highly inflammatory and can contribute to the deterioration of metabolic machinery.

Extra-virgin, cold-pressed, organic olive oil is the way to go because it minimizes processing and the potential to oxidize. Get your oils in dark, glass bottles, as it protects them from both heat and light (and any potential chemicals from plastics). Be sure to store the glass bottle in a cool, dark place.

Refrain from cooking olive oil at high heat: no more than 325°F.

Raw, whole nuts and seeds are also a great source of fat. Macadamia nuts are particularly high in the monounsaturated fat found in avocado and olive oil. Most others are composed primarily of omega 6 fat (walnuts are high in omega 3).

Only consume nuts raw or lightly roasted, and never roasted in oil. The roasting process, whether with oil or dry, creates toxic molecules called *advanced glycation end products* (AGEs, see page 229). You can always purchase raw nuts and season them at home.

Coconut products (oil, meat, cream/milk, and yogurt alternatives) contain a special kind of saturated fat called a medium-chain fatty acid. It boosts brain health and supports a healthy metabolism. Medium-chain fatty acids are stable at high temperatures and so are great for the high-heat cooking you can't do with olive and other plant oils.

Fat doesn't have a designated spot on the Yates Protocol plate because it almost always pairs with something else.

Some fats are great *topping* fats, sprinkled on salads or in stir-fries: nuts, seeds, olives, coconut chips, avocado slices, or hard-boiled egg yolks are all great options. For nuts and seeds, the right portion is half a handful, about 15–20 grams.

Cook your meat, vegetables, or complex carbs/resistant starches in a healthy fat: Ghee or coconut oil are both great options for high-heat cooking.

Finally, dressings, condiments, dips, and sauces often contain fat. If you purchase something store-made, *check the label*. These are typically made with (highly processed and oxidized) seed oils. Sometimes they'll say something like "avocado oil mayonnaise" or "olive oil dressing" on the packaging, but when you look at the nutrition label, it reveals a trick: The healthy fat was added in a small amount just so it could be branded as healthy on the packaging. It's ideal to make these at home.

PRO TIP: BE CAUTIOUS WITH RESTAURANT SAUCES, CURRIES, AND DRESSING

Food prepared at restaurants is almost always a risk because you don't know what's in it. Sauces, curries, and dressings are almost always made with processed seed oils. They also often contain carbohydrates. Even when sauces taste savory, carbohydrates are often hiding in them because carbohydrates like wheat flour, rice flour, tapioca flour, potato flour, dal flour, cornstarch, and others are effective thickeners. One way to tell is by the thickness of the sauce. Another is from the stickiness. Does it drip right off your fork or spoon? Sugar is sticky, so if a sauce clings to your utensils, that's a reliable sign there's carbohydrates in it. A thin and slick sauce can contain sugar, too, but it is less likely. When out at a restaurant and less able to pay close attention and care for your needs, err on the side of caution. You can always ask for sauces on the side.

SWAP THIS FOR THAT

Cheap olive oil in plastic bottles	→	Extra-virgin, cold-pressed, organic olive oil in dark glass bottles
Butter alternatives, margarine, shortening	→	Real, grass-fed butter
Vegetable oil for high-heat cooking	→	Coconut oil or butter
Roasted nuts or seeds	→	Raw nuts or seeds
Deep-fried meat or starch	→	Boiled, steamed, baked, grilled

COMPLEX CARBOHYDRATE/RESISTANT STARCH

Many think carbohydrates are the enemy. Carbohydrates *are* sugar, but you don't need to be afraid of them. You do need to be mindful of how much you eat and the quality.

There are two main categories of carbohydrate: simple and complex.

Simple carbohydrates are the "bad" ones. They are short and uncomplicated, so they pass into the bloodstream lightning quick and take you on a blood-sugar roller coaster. They can really put you up in the sky—and then, bam! Slammed down the other side. This can disrupt mood and cause brain fog and exhaustion. It can also make you feel the need to eat, and especially more simple carbs, even though you're not technically hungry. It can create a cycle of getting on and off the blood-sugar roller coaster, leading to ever-increasing eating and cravings.

Entirely avoid simple carbohydrates at first:

- Added sugars: sugar, syrup, cane syrup, molasses, honey (These are in sweet beverages, desserts, breakfast cereals, and most processed foods—even the savory ones.)

- All white flour from wheat products (These include white bread, white pasta, pizza, cookies, desserts, and pretzels and other snacks.)

- All white rice products

- All flour from other grains

Being cautious around simple carbs means knowing and prioritizing your blood sugar needs. If you're very sensitive and at the beginning of your healing journey, it's best to avoid them entirely. But if you are testing your blood sugar, you may be able to incorporate them if you (1) eat protein or fiber, ideally leafy greens, first, and (2) have only a small portion. Err on the side of caution and go low and slow with your portions. Start with just a quarter of what you'd normally eat. Then, test your blood sugar after. Don't guess. An ideal blood sugar rise after a meal is 20–40, no more than 50, mg/dl.

PRO TIP: EXPERIMENT WITH FOOD ORDER

My patient Raj is a vegetarian who comes from a culture with a lot of curry dishes and rice. I support him in his desire to find a way to make his culture's meals work for him. When we first began working together, his blood sugar spiked after a meal of lentil and vegetable curry with rice. I explained to him that eating protein and/or fiber first can help.

Raj has since found that when his protein source, often lentils or chickpeas, are boiled or prepared only with spices and oil, eating them first is fine for his blood sugar. If he is consuming a meal at a restaurant and there is a thick curry, it can spike his blood sugar. So he tries to order extra leafy greens on the side and eats them before his meal. It makes a difference! If there is rice, naan, or roti, he eats it last and in a small portion. This is how he's made his food preferences and cultural needs work great for his blood sugar journey.

PRO TIP: SOCIAL SITUATIONS

Social life matters. Many people feel anxious or trapped because of the expectations or preferences of friends, workplace, or family members. Sometimes a spouse, partner, parent, or child will refuse to accommodate healthy changes.

My patient Cassandra felt she was in a tough spot. She cooked most of the meals for her spouse and children. Family dinner was important. Her family really liked dishes heavy in simple carbohydrates, and they preferred that fish and chicken be fried. Cassandra didn't want to disappoint anyone, but she also needed to find a way to honor what her body needed.

Cassandra told her spouse and kids: "I'm not judging you for how you eat. I'm not forcing you to eat like me. But I must make some changes to take care of my own health. I think you could benefit from making the change with me, but if you don't want to, now or later, that is okay, too. Let's figure out how we can eat together so everybody feels cared for and is content."

This showed her family that she cared about them while also drawing a boundary about her need to change for her health.

Be firm about what you need.

Complex carbs are the "good" ones. One of my patients calls them "nature's carbs." Nature's carbs are more *complex*, so the gut must break them down into simpler forms before they get absorbed. This slows the move into the bloodstream: with a gentle rise, no big spike, no big drop or crash. They help you avoid cravings, provided you stay within the bounds of eating a certain portion at each meal. Keep complex carbs/resistant starches to 25 percent of your plate.

Complex carbs to include, starting with one cup:

- **Beans, peas, and other legumes.** They contain protein but are mostly carbohydrate.

- **Squashes.** Squashes are vegetables, though they have more carbohydrate than the extra-fibrous leafy greens. A medium zucchini contains just 6 grams of carbs. Sweeter varieties like butternut squash have more.

- **Potatoes, sweet potatoes, yams, and other tubers.** These are nutrient-rich sources of complex carbohydrates, especially if you keep the skin on.

Complex carbs to potentially include, starting with half a slice or a cup:

- **Whole grains.** These qualify as complex carbohydrates, but as stated above, you must be cautious. A half cup of pasta or half slice of bread is a good portion to begin with. You must also be cautious regarding food sensitivities. Many people have grain intolerance. Not just gluten.

- Brown, black, wild, jasmine, and other rice with the fiber jacket firmly in place. Like whole grains, these qualify as complex carbohydrates but require caution.

- **Quinoa.** It's a seed that is mostly complex carbohydrate, with some protein in it.

- **Fruit.** Fruit is technically a complex carbohydrate, but it's high in sugar. Our culture has a myth: You must eat five servings of fruit a day to meet your vitamin requirements. The truth is, most of the vitamins found in fruit are also found in vegetables, and in higher quantities. For example, broccoli contains more vitamin C than oranges. You don't need to get a certain amount of fruit in your diet, or any fruit at all. But fruit can be a healthful source of complex carbohydrate, especially if it's fibrous. Berries are the best because they contain the most antioxidants and fiber. With other fruits like apples and peaches, leave the skin on. No peeling!

Fruit juice is 100 percent no.

Finally, there is a special kind of complex carbohydrate known as a resistant starch. All complex carbohydrates have at least a little resistant starch, but some special ones have significant amounts.

Include resistant starch as much as possible. Like fiber, resistant starch is indigestible by humans, but there are important, gut-protecting bacteria all the way at the end of the digestive tract that love to eat it. This is where the name comes from: It *resists* digestion until the very end. Feeding these end-of-the-line bacteria is excellent for helping heal type 2 and prediabetes as well as many other conditions. It helps with blood sugar management, lowering bad cholesterol, supporting insulin sensitivity, improving the gut's microbiome, and controlling appetite and weight.

Cool down your starches. As starch in food cools down, some become resistant. This is the case for rice, grains, white potatoes, sweet potatoes, yams, and other tubers like jicama, cassava, beets, parsnips, turnips, yucca, and rutabaga. You don't have to eat it cold. You can reheat the food again after cooling. Remain cautious with the portion. Turning rice, potatoes, or a grain product into a more resistant starch is health-promoting but won't necessarily reduce the blood sugar response too much. See how you respond. Test, don't guess!

Highest resistant starch foods:

Green bananas (including the peels) and green banana flour

Plantains

Chicory root

Oats

Beans, peas, and other legumes

White potatoes, if cooked and then cooled

Rice and grains, if cooked and then cooled

Sweet potatoes, yams, and other tubers like jicama, cassava, beets, turnips, parsnips, yucca, and rutabaga, if cooked and then cooled

Nuts and seeds, while not complex carbs, also contain small amounts of resistant starch.

SWAP THIS FOR THAT

Yellow bananas →	Green bananas
Yellow bananas →	Plantains
White rice →	Cooled white rice
White rice →	Cooled brown or other whole rice
Freshly cooked potatoes & other root vegetables →	Cooled potatoes & other root vegetables

HYDRATION

Almost all drinks that aren't water or plain tea are sweetened with sugar or sugar substitutes. Avoid all juice, sweet tea, coffee with any added sweet tastes (whether natural or artificial), soda, and diet soda—100 percent avoid.

One glass of orange juice contains three whole oranges. Companies often advertise something like "contains three servings of fruit!" on the label. This is not a good thing—that's a lot of sugar without any of the fiber that would come with eating the actual fruit. Three whole oranges contain about 36 grams of naturally occurring sugar. And that's just for juice with "no sugar added."

If you've found something you think might be an exception to these rules, pay very close attention to the ingredient lists and the serving size. Any fruit juice in the ingredient list is basically all sugar. If you do drink a beverage like this, notice how you feel afterward. If you feel sleepy, tired, brain-fogged, or are struggling to focus, your body is telling you that this "juice" is dragging you on a blood-sugar roller-coaster ride.

We also need to square with serving sizes.

When I was a child, we drank juice out of specific juice glasses, and they were 4 ounces. How big are glasses for children and adults today? Too big!

For most drinks today, the standard serving size on the nutrition label is "one cup." One cup is 8 fluid ounces, which is two-thirds the size of a can of soda, or one-half the size of a typical plastic bottle.

If you drink one glass of soda, juice, or sweet tea all at once, you'll have a blood sugar spike, guaranteed. If you drink one or more glasses slowly over the course of the day, you'll have chronically elevated blood sugar and insulin, guaranteed. One cup is too much, no matter how you drink it.

What about diet soda? Artificial sweeteners? Also 100 percent no. Why? It's true that they have no calories, no "real" sugar. This sounds good in theory . . . but these can cause major problems. They confuse the link between the tongue and the brain. They increase cravings. People who consume artificially sweetened drinks typically end up with stronger cravings and the consumption of more calories later. Artificial sweeteners can also cause insulin levels to rise even in the absence of real sugar. They feed bad bacteria in the gut, crowd out the good bacteria in the gut's microbiome, creating uncomfortable digestive problems like gas and contributing to inflammation, pain, immune system problems, insulin resistance, and type 2 diabetes.

Two natural sweeteners, stevia and monk fruit, which are derived from plants, may be okay in moderation. But watch your blood sugar and pay attention to your cravings.

SWAP THIS:

Soda
Diet soda
Fruit juice
Vegetable juice
Sweet tea
Any sweetened beverage

FOR THAT:

Unsweetened herbal tea
Green tea
Sparkling water aka carbonated or mineral water
You can add strawberries, cucumber, ginger, peppermint, or spices for flavor.

Eight 8- or 10-ounce glasses of water a day is ideal. If you exercise a lot, live in a hot or dry place, or sweat a lot for any reason, you'll need more. If you take prescription medications, check with your doctor to see if they have a higher water demand and you require more water.

PRO TIP: KEEP AN EYE ON CAFFEINE

Caffeine can stimulate a blood sugar response. The amount is different for everyone. If you drink caffeinated beverages, test your blood sugar after to see if you have a response. Caffeine can also stimulate the release of cortisol, the stress hormone, and create feelings of being wired or anxious. It can exacerbate stress and can disrupt sleep, especially if you drink it later in the day. Pay attention to how you feel up to eight hours after drinking caffeine.

BREAKFAST

It's the same Yates Protocol template: 50 percent vegetables with a focus on leafy greens, 25 percent lean protein, and 25 percent complex carbs/resistant starch, with healthy fats incorporated as needed.

Every meal should be savory and start with leafy greens or another vegetable—*even breakfast.*

Many think breakfast foods must be sweet. American breakfasts *used* to be savory: eggs, bacon, sausages, potatoes, butter. Sweet breakfast took over because food companies figured out how addictive a hit of sugar can be in the morning.

Steak, fish, beans, vegetables, for breakfast? Yes! Start eating them at breakfast and you may realize savory breakfast feels right for you.

Lean protein is very important at breakfast: Eat a few eggs or some slices of meat, steak, turkey bacon, or salmon. Eat it first. Lean protein gives your body the important building blocks it needs to tackle the rest of your day head-on. It helps keep you satisfied and energized throughout the day. You can add some chickpeas or lentils to your eggs for a blood-sugar-friendly nutrient boost.

Healthy fats are also important for getting your blood sugar off on the right foot! Eggs, fatty fish, or half an avocado are excellent early-morning fat sources.

Do you like smoothies for breakfast? Be careful. If purchasing from the store or an online retailer, scrutinize the ingredient list. It's usually best to make your own.

PRO TIP: GIVE SAVORY BREAKFAST A CHANCE, LIKE JORGE

My patient Jorge was in the habit of having sweet breakfast, specifically cereal, instant oatmeal, and granola. Sometimes he ate bagels or muffins, or when out for breakfast he'd eat a croissant or baked good with his coffee. Our culture has a widespread myth (promulgated by food companies) that breakfast cereal, instant oatmeal, granola, muffins, etc., are good for you. But they're almost always not.

I suggested he commit to savory breakfast for two weeks.

Jorge chose huevos rancheros, a breakfast dish he had once enjoyed eating with his grandmother.

At the end of two weeks, Jorge told me he couldn't believe how much more energy he had during the day, how much his blood sugar numbers improved, and that he no longer had urges to snack in the afternoon. He started experimenting with new savory breakfast options: omelets with vegetables and salsa, eggs scrambled with black beans or other legumes, steak and eggs cooked over easy, smoked salmon with poached eggs. The possibilities are truly endless.

LUNCH

Do not skip it!

Just as with breakfast, fill your plate with fibrous vegetables, lean protein, healthy fat, and some complex carbs/resistant starch.

DINNER

For dinner, it's the same template and ratios. If you're going to eat one meal lower carbohydrate, make it this one to help your body reset blood sugar overnight. It's also best to say no to fruit for your source of complex carbs/resistant starch.

DESSERT

It's best not to have dessert, period. If you have a craving for something sweet, fresh fruit is the best option. Never have dessert first, ever. It'll zap your blood sugar right up.

PRO TIP: GIVE YOUR GUT 15 MINUTES TO LET YOU KNOW IF YOU HAD ENOUGH TO EAT

Commit to appropriate portions of food for each meal. Once you've eaten the amount of food you committed to, wait fifteen minutes. Many people get distracted by the TV or their phones and don't notice they are overeating. Portions are very important for blood sugar management. Give your gut and brain a chance to communicate. If you're no longer hungry after fifteen minutes, it's time to stop eating.

PRO TIP: FLOSS AND BRUSH

Floss and brush your teeth right after that last meal of the day. It's a powerful signal to your brain that you are done eating and helps combat the feeling that treats or snacks are calling to you between meals.

MEAL SWAPS—THERE'S A WAY!

The kitchen is a wonderful place to flex your creativity. If you love apple pie, what about a few slices of apple with walnuts and cinnamon? If you love cereal or granola, an unsweetened almond or coconut yogurt with nuts and some slices of fruit is an excellent swap. If you love pumpkin pie, try pureeing pumpkin or butternut squash with pumpkin pie spice and serving it with unsweetened almond or coconut yogurt, or spread the puree on a small slice of whole grain toast with butter. The possibilities are endless.

SUCCESSFUL FORAGING: HOW TO IDENTIFY AND BUY HEALTHY FOODS

The grocery store is the modern forest or jungle. Dangers lurk on every shelf. Is a food *healthy*? How can you tell? Today, trillion-dollar industries pay food scientists top dollar to make the sweetest, saltiest, tastiest foods as addictive as possible, with the cheapest ingredients, and then sell them to us as "healthy." This is a whole new ball game.

Particularly with desserts, snacks, fast food, candy bars: The science of it is stunning. People's brains light up as if they had cocaine, alcohol, or opioids. You get deeply rewarded by these foods. Not satisfied. Rewarded. Pleasure centers get triggered. Your brain can't forget. You can't wait until the next time. It's a precise science of intentional addiction.

The companies that peddle these addictive products also pay advertisers top dollar to make the most persuasive ads and packaging possible. Typically, they design it to deceive us. Almost everything on grocery store shelves is optimized for profit . . . at the expense of our health.

We have to fight back, and we have to be smart with our choices. In the grocery store, the best way to avoid toxic foods is to buy fresh from the produce and meat sections. Except for some cooking oils and spices, you can in theory do all your shopping only in these sections of the grocery store.

It *is* possible to find prepared foods and sauces, frozen meals, and the like that are healthy. There *is* a small but growing number of health-conscious food companies in the world. But how do you know which are which?

Start by making sure you aren't duped by any packaging gimmicks.

Here is a list of common red flags on food packaging:

"LOW FAT"

When a label proclaims a food is low or reduced fat, sugar is often added. It's also often highly processed. In general, full-fat versions of foods are better for blood sugar management.

"HEART HEALTHY"

Advertisers put this on packaging for many reasons, usually because the product is relatively lower in saturated fat or high in fiber or grains. Neither of these things necessarily make a product healthy or good for your blood sugar management.

"NO ADDED SUGAR!"

No added sugar means there is *already* sugar in the product. This is a common claim on fruit juices. Sugar can be sky-high without any added sugar.

"ZERO SUGAR!"

If the packaging of a sweet food claims there is zero sugar, then it almost surely contains sugar substitutes, which can harm health and increase cravings.

"JUST X GRAMS OF SUGAR PER SERVING!"

If the packaging advertises a low amount of sugar *per serving*, it's possibly because the serving size is very small. Make sure you assess how much sugar there is per portion.

NUTRITION LABELS: HOW TO AVOID BEING TRICKED

Nutrition labels have three key elements you must look at. From top to bottom, it's 1: the serving size; 2: the macronutrient breakdown; and 3: the most important part—the ingredient list, in tiny print, down at the very bottom.

Macronutrient breakdown:

The total amount of fat, protein, and carbohydrate in every serving is listed on the label in the box of lined rows, with some subcategories. For fat, there are the subcategories trans fat and saturated fat. For carbohydrate, there are subcategories for added sugar and fiber. Remember: This is *per serving*.

The rows for "trans fat" and sugar are deceptive. A company can list "0 grams" of either if the amount per serving is 0.4 grams or less (it rounds down to zero).

To spot trans fat or sugar in any food, you *must* look at the ingredient list. Watch for margarine, shortening, partially hydrogenated or hydrogenated oils.

The same goes for sugar. A company can list "0 grams" of sugar or added sugar if the amount per serving is 0.4 grams or less.

Sometimes diabetes books recommend subtracting the "fiber" from the "total carbohydrates" because fiber is digested by gut bacteria more than by you. They call this "net carbs." But this is getting in the weeds. Start with small portions and always test, don't guess.

Ingredient list:

The ingredient list is the most important part of any food label, despite being as hidden as possible.

If an ingredient list is very long or contains a word your grand-mother wouldn't recognize, be wary. You may just want to put it right back on the shelf. This suggests the food in your hand is highly processed and has been designed to make you addicted to it, not to support your health.

Then dive deeper. Ingredient lists always go in order of "most" to "least." The first ingredient is the most prominent, followed by the second, and on and on.

There are a few major tricks to look out for:

False promises: Sometimes a product will promise a specific ingredient on the packaging. For example, many condiment companies sell an Olive Oil Hummus. The term "Olive Oil Hummus" is meant to make you think you're about to purchase a hummus made with chickpeas and olive oil. *Nope.* It almost always *isn't.* Olive oil is *included*, but usually only a small amount. If one of the first ingredients is a different oil, such as soybean oil—and olive oil is listed *after* it or even near the end of the ingredient list, that means the hummus is made primarily of soybean oil.

Sugar sneaking: Often, companies use sugar in different forms to break up the total amount into smaller bits. This saves them from having to list sugar as the first ingredient. For example, the ingredient list of a breakfast cereal might say "enriched wheat flour, malt syrup, barley syrup, high-fructose corn syrup." . . . Guess what. Ingredients 2, 3, and 4 are all different kinds of sugar.

Watch out for any ingredient that ends in "ose." It's a sugar: fructose, dextrose, glucose, maltose, lactose, high-fructose corn syrup, sucrose, maltose. There is also cane juice, evaporated cane juice, cane syrup, cane sugar, corn sweetener, corn syrup, corn syrup solids, barley malt, malt sugar, malt syrup, invert sugar, raw sugar, turbinado. Any "syrup" is a sugar. Honey, agave, molasses: all sugars. Fruit juice concentrate is also a sugar.

Sugar substitutes: Sometimes packaging will say "zero sugar." If it's a sweet food, your alarm bells should ring. There's probably a sugar substitute.

Sugar substitutes include: aspartame (NutraSweet, Equal), acesulfame potassium (Sweet One, Sunett), neotame (Newtame), saccharin (Sweet'n Low), sucralose (Splenda).

Stevia and monk fruit are natural, plant-based sugar substitutes, but may not have the same negative impact as other sugar substitutes.

Natural flavors: In the USA, a very large number of chemicals, including MSG (monosodium glutamate), which may contribute to many health conditions including anxiety, migraines, and insomnia, are permitted to be lumped together under "natural flavors." If you want to be wary of processing chemicals and additives, steer clear of "natural flavors."

Calories per serving: There is one other part of nutrition labels I haven't mentioned: the calories. I'm mentioning it last because it's the least important part. It's the least important part because the *quality* of what you eat matters a whole lot more than the quantity.

Calories are listed at the top of the label. It's the biggest and most obvious part of the whole label on purpose. It diverts attention from the ingredient list, that is, the processed and toxic ingredients they use to try to make us addicted to their products. Reclaim your agency and health. Focus on the ingredient list.

SHOULD YOU COUNT CALORIES?

Generally, I do not recommend counting calories. It's important to have good portion control for managing blood sugar. But my patients naturally eat appropriate portions when they switch to nourishing foods and support healthy sleep, reduce stress, time meals right, and exercise. Sometimes it takes more in-depth emotional work or gut bacteria healing to restore proper appetite signaling, but it can happen naturally. Healing and eating nutritious food are the most sustainable way to achieve healthy portion control.

For people with visceral fat in the abdomen around the organs, i.e., belly fat, losing weight can typically help with type 2 and prediabetes. Nitpicking how much you eat can be a recipe for yo-yo dieting, low self-esteem, frustration, and giving up. Counting calories can be helpful for some people. Some do it in an emotionally healthy way that helps them understand portions. Talk with a health-care practitioner you trust about the best approach for you.

ON A BUDGET

My favorite tips for eating healthy on a budget include going local, shopping what's in season, buying in bulk, watching holiday deals, and checking the freezer aisle.

Shop local: Grass-fed, pasture-raised animal products and organic produce are more expensive up front but can be cost-effective because they're more satiating. Beyond that, you can be even more cost-effective if you buy them locally. Look for local farms or Community Supported Agriculture (CSA) programs.

Shop seasonal: Local produce is often less expensive than that found in grocery stores shipped in from around the globe. This means you eat foods in season, since you get the produce right when it's growing from the ground. Many areas have growing networks of local, smaller farms. They often have centralized markets, newsletters, or even distributors that are constantly hunting for good deals. Farmers markets can be excellent for finding great produce at great prices.

If your budget forces you to choose between local and organic, choose local. Many local farms simply don't have the resources to get certified as organic, and often, larger farms can get certified but don't participate in the highest-quality sustainability practices.

Shop in bulk: Sometimes purchasing in bulk isn't the panacea it's made it out to be. When you buy in bulk you have to spend more up front. Some of us can't do that. Consider going in on it with a neighbor or friend. Look for dry beans, peas, chickpeas, and lentils as they have a long shelf life. Do the math to be sure buying in bulk is actually cost saving.

Shop holiday deals: For nonperishable goods—such as coconut oil, olive oil, bulk beans, peas, and other legumes, condiments, or anything dried, canned, or frozen, you can help your budget by waiting for big sale days. Black Friday, Cyber Monday, post-Christmas, New Year's, etc.

Shop frozen: Frozen produce is typically flash frozen right off the vine, preserving its nutrients. Frozen berries will likely have more nutrients than a pint of berries shipped from the other side of the world. Plus, having frozen foods on hand is a great way to make sure you've got healthy options if you can't get out to go shopping.

Don't cut budget corners on healthy fats: One corner you don't want to cut is highly processed cooking oils. They're easy to spot because they're super cheap, come in large quantities, and are in clear plastic bottles. Invest in dark, glass bottles and extra-virgin, organic, cold-pressed oils.

It might also be better for your budget to buy foods from specific ethnic markets that cater to Latino, African, Asian, Caribbean, South Asian, Indian, or Mediterranean cuisines.

PRO TIP: GIVE YOURSELF 3–4 WEEKS TO ADAPT YOUR TASTE BUDS

After years or a lifetime of eating the ultra-processed food designed to hijack your taste buds and send your pleasure centers into a frenzy, fresh foods can be a shock to the system. If your tongue isn't used to these more subtle flavors, it can take 10–14 days to adjust the taste buds and how they communicate with the brain. Your taste buds turn over for a fresh set every 10–14 days. Be patient. Don't expect this to shift overnight.

FINDING WHICH FOODS FROM THE YATES PROTOCOL TEMPLATE ARE BEST FOR YOU

Individuals have unique responses to foods. To find the best foods for you and have the most success managing your individual blood sugar, it is crucial to test, not to guess.

The basic idea is simple: Use the foods I've listed in this chapter, in the portions I describe, as your template. Pick ones you enjoy! Then, monitor your blood sugar, and get curious about any unusual spikes you experience. Use the gift of data from your continuous glucose monitor (or glucometer) to keep looking for ways to heal your metabolic machinery while bringing your blood sugar responses to meals down, and down, and down.

THE WHATABOUTS

Nutrition is complex. You may be wondering about a few common questions. Here are the most common "but what about . . ." questions I receive.

What about dairy?

For most people, about 85 percent of my patients, there is some kind of dairy intolerance. This usually means spikes in blood sugar along with some common symptoms, such as upset stomach, constantly runny nose, sniffles, constipation or diarrhea, skin problems, chronic ear infections, and more.

Sometimes people continue eating dairy products even though they have symptoms. But these symptoms are only the ones you can see on the surface. What else is silently happening beneath? Get to know your body. Honor what it needs.

The few 25–35 percent (estimates vary: 36 percent, 24 percent) of people in the world most likely to be able to tolerate dairy are people of Central and Northern European descent, as well as from subcultures in the Middle East, in North Africa, and some in South Asia. About 80 percent of African and Native Americans and 90 percent of Asian Americans are likely intolerant. Those from most Asian, most African, and Central and South American cultures are highly unlikely to tolerate dairy well.

Most don't tolerate dairy well because the proteins in cow's milk are large. Milk proteins are the smallest in human breast milk, followed by sheep and goat. Cow's milk proteins are the biggest. Being big matters because the bigger the protein, the harder it is for the immune system to manage. If you let children wean by themselves, they stop consuming breast milk before they turn five years old. The small intestine stops being able to deal with the proteins in milk naturally. Why force your body to process something it no longer wants or needs?

If you want to experiment with dairy, you must test. You can try different categories of dairy. You could have different reactions to milk, yogurt, hard cheese, soft cheese, and this may vary across dairy from cows, sheep, or goats. These foods *can* be very nutrient-rich, especially the full-fat versions.

Dairy has the three normal macronutrients in it: fat, protein, and carbohydrates. The parts that are most often trouble for health are the proteins (casein and whey) and carbohydrate (lactose). Yogurt and milk contain all three macronutrients: fat, protein, and carbohydrates. Cream contains all three, too, though is especially high in fat. Cheese is all fat and protein, no carbs. Sometimes people tolerate hard and soft cheeses differently due to the different protein content. Butter is almost pure fat: 99 percent fat with trace amounts of casein and whey. Ghee is purified butter, stripped of the trace proteins. It's 100 percent fat.

Watch your blood sugar for at least 120 minutes.

Today there are some excellent alternatives to dairy. Almond, cashew, and coconut products are delicious. They're processed, but more minimally. Be sure to check the label. Sugar and sugar alternatives are often added, so choose unsweetened varieties.

What about alcohol?

I recommend against alcohol for blood sugar management, but some varieties have lower impacts than others. Be sure to consume at least 3–5 hours before bed. If drinking alcohol, pass on juice or other sweetened mixers, beer, and sweet wine. Red wine could be tolerated decently, especially if made with non-GMO yeast, and is high in antioxidants. Spirits are lower in carbohydrate and might be tolerated in small portions. If you consume multiple drinks, no more than one an hour, and two in total. Monitor your blood sugar during this time and again the next day, as there can be a significant effect hours later. Eating food before drinking alcohol, in the recommended order of protein and fiber (leafy greens) first, might help moderate the impact of alcohol on blood sugar levels.

What about condiments or dressing?

Read the labels. Watch serving size. Beware of "low fat" and "low calorie" versions. Mustard is typically well tolerated. Ketchup and barbecue sauce are usually very high in sugar. If you use ketchup or barbecue condiments, use them sparingly and count them as a source of simple carbohydrate.

Mayonnaise is typically all fat. It is often made with processed vegetable oil, so scrutinize the label. Look for versions made with avocado, MCT (medium-chain triglyceride), or olive oil, and check the label to make sure it's the primary fat. Keep an eye out for added sugar, too. "Low fat" mayonnaise or dressing typically has added sugar or some other shenanigans to make up for the reduced fat quantity.

What about fermented foods?

Fermented foods contain live bacteria cultures and are a bonus for your gut microbiome.

Excellent fermented foods include kimchi, sauerkraut, pickles (watch out for added salt), beets, and carrots. These can be homemade. If you purchase them in the store, make sure they have live bacteria cultures. Some on the shelf are designed to taste fermented but have no live cultures.

What about dark chocolate?

Dark chocolate and raw cacao are often well tolerated, especially if there's no added sugar. Remember that chocolate and cacao have caffeine. Check the labels and go with small portions.

In this chapter, you learned:

- There are four basic food groups: fiber, lean protein, healthy fats, and complex carbs/resistant starches. Each food group provides important nourishment that helps you heal.

- Build every plate with:

  - 50 percent high-fiber vegetables, with a focus on leafy greens,

  - 25 percent lean protein,

  - 25 percent complex carbohydrate/resistant starch.

- Hydrate only with water and unsweetened tea.

- At the grocery, focus on fresh produce and always read nutrition labels, with the understanding that processed foods are designed to addict you and their labels to trick you.

- Every time you eat is an opportunity for healing. Take advantage of it!

Quick wins/first steps:

- Add leafy greens to dinner 7 days a week.

- Swap soda and sweetened beverages for water and unsweetened teas.

- Swap deep-fried foods for grilled or sauteed foods.

- Swap rice for cauliflower rice, and grain noodles for zucchini noodles.

- Have a savory, protein-rich breakfast every morning.

- Identify major obstacles to eating well at home, the office, or on the road and find ways to overcome them.

CHAPTER 2

Meal Timing

Use This Scientifically Proven Eating Rhythm to
Improve Cravings, Energy, and Blood Sugar Control

CHAPTER MAP

This chapter explains a basic eating rhythm that heals
metabolic damage and offers intermittent fasting to
accelerate healing.

KEY SECTIONS

- The basic rhythm
- Lunch is self-care . . . Never skip it!
- The twin gremlins of appetite: ghrelin and leptin
- Snacking: don't, but if you do . . .
- Intermittent fasting: Timed Windows for Healing

*Maria worked very hard running an amazing Italian restaurant
with her husband. She arrived before breakfast and stayed until*

11 p.m. *This was impressive, but it also involved a lot of unintentional compromises of Maria's health.*

She had high blood pressure, bad cholesterol, sleep apnea, GERD, type 2 diabetes, obesity, and other chronic illnesses. She was struggling. She decided to tackle meal timing first on the Yates Protocol.

Part of Maria's job meant she never sat down to eat a meal. She snacked all day. She hadn't considered this a problem and had even heard that eating six small meals throughout the day "stokes metabolic fires." She and her husband had a big dinner after closing the restaurant around 11 p.m. Their go-to dish was fettuccine Alfredo.

We moved her dinnertime to 6 p.m. It helped reduce her cravings and give her more natural hunger ebbs and flows. It improved her energy and blood sugar balance. It unlocked her ability to take the reins and inch by inch, step by step, implement the rest.

Meal timing is such a gift. It's such a gift and almost no one talks about it. The body works best on its natural rhythm: in meals earlier in the day, never late at night. It needs this natural rhythm for healthy blood sugar balance. If you eat outside that, you're forcing your body to fight an uphill battle. All the time.

Maria had always felt hungry, that feeling of I could eat, *all day long, and then starving in the evening, so she ate that huge plate of pasta. This isn't what you want. You want* Now I'm hungry, now I'm full, now I'm hungry, now I'm full *starting in the morning. I helped Maria implement the natural rhythm her body was craving: hearty breakfast, hearty lunch, moderate dinner. No more snacking. It restored the natural ebb and flow of her appetite. She reclaimed a degree of mental clarity and energy around food she hadn't even really known she'd lost. It also helped her metabolism. Her energy went up, and her blood sugar levels improved. She made peace with food.*

EATING RIGHT MEANS AT THE RIGHT TIME

Eating right means eating the right food—but also *at the right time*. This is a crucial element our culture often overlooks.

The body has a natural rhythm. It has times it likes to fuel up, times it likes to burn that fuel, and times it likes to rest and reset for the next day.

Meal timing is the art and science of using this natural rhythm to your advantage. Get in harmony with the rhythms your body is made for, and you get natural energy. You support your metabolism. You heal the cellular damage driving blood sugar and insulin dysregulation.

THE BODY RUNS ON CELLULAR CLOCKS

It's easy to forget, living in today's concrete and fluorescent jungles, but we are natural beings, born to operate according to the rhythms of the earth. There's night, day, summer, and winter. Every day the sun rises, and ecosystems wake up. We are natural beings made to be in natural harmony with these rhythms. Every cell in the body keeps track of time. Remarkable, but true! It performs its functions on a schedule.

The overall rhythm of the body is the *circadian rhythm*. It's regulated by information from many sources. The biggest regulator is the light in the sky. Light is detected by a part of the brain called the thalamus, which sends a signal to other cells about what time it is. How much time do you spend outdoors? It matters.

The second most influential factor is when you eat. Your body expects you to eat in a certain rhythm. If you honor this rhythm, then you give yourself a wonderful gift. Eat the right amount of food at the right time and you help cells do their job. You help them burn energy and use and store sugar efficiently. Eat at the wrong time and you confuse them. They get less efficient storing blood sugar and resetting blood sugar levels. Start working with and supporting the natural rhythm with meal timing, and you'll improve appetite, sleep, energy, weight, fasting blood sugar, fasting insulin, and A1C.

THE BASIC RHYTHM

The ideal, basic eating pattern for most people with type 2 or prediabetes:

3 meals a day, spaced 4–5 hours apart, and concluding 3–5 hours before bedtime

Breakfast or lunch is the biggest meal. Dinner is the smallest. If you are intermittent fasting, you can skip breakfast and have a bigger lunch, or follow the guidance intended for the type of intermittent fasting you are doing or your doctor's guidance.

No snacks.

That's it! It's simple, but so powerful.

This basic rhythm:

- provides enough time between meals for blood sugar and other metabolic processes to reset before the next meal,

- fills you up enough to prevent the need to snack,

- provides enough time to digest before sleep and overnight while your body resets blood sugar and insulin sensitivity.

There is flexibility depending on your needs. If you wake at 7:00 a.m., you could have breakfast at 7:30, 8:00, or 9:00, for example. Just make sure you wait about 4–5 hours before lunch, and again before dinner. If intermittent fasting, you can delay breakfast or skip breakfast and have lunch at 11:00 or 12:00. Leave at least 3–5 hours between dinner and bed. Then, be consistent with it.

THE IMPORTANCE OF EATING MEALS EARLIER IN THE DAY

Why bigger meals earlier in the day? Imagine living out in nature. No fast food, no frozen pizzas, no food delivery apps. There are not even grocery stores, or kitchens with electricity. What would you do? When would you eat?

Without refrigeration, you'd have to eat most meals fresh. That means cooking right before you eat. There also wasn't artificial lighting, so you'd cook when the sun was out. Cooking would be laborious, so you would do it two or three times a day at most. You'd have to clean up after each meal, and you'd also have to make sure food was safely put away for the night—you wouldn't want bears prowling around looking for your food!—so you'd stop eating well before the sun set. You usually wouldn't be able to prepare anything overnight.

We have all but forgotten these natural rhythms and elements of life. We got out of sync in a few major ways.

Many of us are chronic snackers. Premade, processed food is available to us 24 hours a day, 7 days a week: chips in the pantry, candy at the checkout counter, trail mix in the car. Convenience stores and fast-food restaurants are on every corner, with flashing signs, some even pumping odors into the air to entice you to go in. Many of us are almost never without food: eating it all day long, and late at night, when we're not supposed to, usually more later in the day after work has ended and we're melting into the sofa.

If you snack all the time, you never get properly hungry and you never get properly full, either. The body has powerful hormones it uses to signal hunger and fullness. But those require eating in meals. You end up constantly feeling like you need to eat, and also like it's never enough.

Some people are *go go go* and don't eat enough early in the day. Many subsist on coffee or energy drinks—which have no nutrition in them, and usually tons of sugar. By the end of a day like this, you're super hungry. Your body has been trying to get you to eat a nutritious meal all day. Your hunger signals are through the roof. You might snarf down your meal in just a few minutes. You'll eat more than you normally would because you're just *that* hungry.

One way or the other, people eat most of their calories at the end of the day, when least active and nearing bedtime. This is a real recipe for metabolic chaos. You leave your body too much work to do while you sleep. This is when it wants to reset blood sugar—but you've given it a lot of digesting to do first. You've delayed the natural cleanup processes. It's like turning off the dishwasher before it's done because you started it too late. You don't get to clean up the way you're designed. You wake up with higher blood sugar numbers than you would otherwise, and often feel less well rested. It's a bad start to the day.

Big, late dinners and late-night snacking are associated with metabolic disorders, insulin resistance, and heightened risk of heart disease. In contrast, hearty early meals and earlier dinners have been shown to improve morning blood sugar and A1C.

What about cultures where people eat late at night? Cultures where people eat late at night often eat real food all day. Because they eat real food, perhaps in these cultural contexts, eating late is not a problem. These cultures also tend to be calmer. They're not living with so much pervasive stress.

Give your organs a chance to repair and restore while asleep. Give your cells the gift of the right signals at the right times. Your body will reward you: increased energy, better mood, better appetite regulation, more efficient metabolic processes, easier weight control, and no blood sugar rockets or cliffs.

EAT ENOUGH AT EVERY MEAL

An important part of the daily rhythm is eating *enough* at every meal—but also not too much. Portions play a big role in blood sugar.

If too big, they can put you on that blood-sugar roller coaster; if too small, you can develop difficulties with hunger and appetite.

If you find yourself routinely getting excessively hungry in the five-hour window before dinner, try eating more at lunch. You want to be hungry before your next meal but not so much that you start feeling obsessive or hangry (a combo of "hungry" and "angry").

LUNCH IS SELF-CARE . . . NEVER SKIP IT!

The biggest and most common mistake I see people make is skipping lunch.

Lunch sets you up for success. It keeps you in the rhythm and helps you stay in control of your choices later. Skipping lunch makes you hungry and hangry. Your hunger signals get stronger and stronger. You become more likely to snack during the afternoon, or to indulge in the most convenient—and not necessarily most healthy— foods later.

Pressed for time when lunch rolls around? Stressed about finding a healthy option? The secret is planning. Preparing lunch ahead of time is self-care. Always bring lunch with you, whether you plan to be at work, running errands, or anywhere else.

NAVIGATING THE OFFICE OR OUT-AND-ABOUT

If coworkers are ordering takeout and you must participate, stick to what you know you can handle. Order familiar healthy foods. Pick according to the four food groups as best as you are able. Get sauces and dressings on the side or ditch them altogether. Ask to have your hamburger on a lettuce wrap and ditch the bun. Choose baked, grilled, or steamed options. Restaurants usually serve overly big portions. You can always stick to the appetizer menu, get a few sides, or save the leftovers for dinner.

Yet you don't have to stress like this. Preparation helps. Give yourself the gift of a healthy lunch. Bring what you need.

As a little girl, I watched my mother meal prep every weekend. As I grew older, I helped with meal preparation and cooking. Now, looking back, I see the wisdom in what she taught me. I invite you to batch cook on weekends. Make five lunches every weekend. Once every month or so you can make some extra stew or soup and put it in the freezer for emergencies. Then, every day of the week, you can take a healthy meal with you—no matter where you're going.

PRO TIP: MEAL PREP ON THE WEEKENDS

My patient Robert worked in an office environment where everybody always went out for lunch or ordered takeout. Robert told me he hadn't thought it was a problem for his blood sugar. "I always order the healthy options!"

But his blood sugar numbers weren't improving.

Most people severely underestimate how much sugar, refined flour, other simple carbs, unhealthy fat, and salt is in the food they order from restaurants. You don't get informed of this on purpose. Restaurant food is typically jam-packed with ingredients designed to prioritize taste (and often profit).

When you make your meals in your own kitchen, *you decide.* You know what you're putting in your body. *You* have control over your blood sugar. Convinced by these ideas, Robert decided to give meal prep a chance.

Robert committed to bringing his own meals to work for at least two weeks. He stopped getting "hangry" before dinner, felt more able to make healthy choices about what to eat, and didn't feel as beholden to dessert or mindless munching while watching TV, especially at night. He also had more predictable and stable blood sugar. Over time, his

A1C began coming down, too. These were all major wins. Robert's co-workers understood and didn't put any pressure on him as he had worried they might. Turns out some of them were ready for a change, too.

CRASHING IN THE AFTERNOON?

Cortisol is the main hormone responsible for keeping you awake and alert. It naturally dips a bit in the midafternoon. Even with this dip, your energy should be good and steady throughout the afternoon. Good sleep and meal timing support that. If you're doing a face-plant on your desk or falling asleep in your chair after lunch, something is taking you on that blood sugar roller-coaster ride and causing it to bottom out in the low, potentially hypoglycemic range.

Monitor your blood sugar numbers in the afternoon. Are they crashing? Are they spiking?

It could be what you're eating for lunch. Are you filling your plate with leafy greens? Do you have a palm-size portion of protein and some healthy fat? How much and which type of carbohydrate are you consuming? Monitor blood sugar for two hours after your meal. If you're crashing in the afternoon, it could be something you're eating a few hours before.

There are other potential sources of afternoon tiredness. Both poor sleep and chronic stress drain you and make you more likely to crash in the afternoon. If you can't identify a plausible cause, it could be mitochondrial insufficiency or some other physiological damage that you can help heal with mitochondrial support. Mitochondria are often exhausted by metabolic damage. This forces both you and your cells to try to operate with little natural energy. I recommend talking to your doctor. I recommend specific supplements for this support; check out the Resources section on my website for more information.

THE TWIN GREMLINS OF APPETITE: GHRELIN AND LEPTIN

Many hormones play a role in the symphony of the body's eating rhythm, but the two most important ones are ghrelin and leptin. I call them the twin gremlins because they are small but powerful. Like gremlins, they can cause a lot of trouble if out of whack! Ghrelin is the main hormone that signals hunger. You can remember it by thinking of the stomach growling—it sounds like "growling," which is similar to how the word *ghrelin* is pronounced. Leptin is the main hormone that signals you are no longer hungry: You've had enough to eat, and it is time to stop eating. Leptin signals satiety, the feeling of being satisfied with what you ate.

When you skip lunch, or snack, or eat late at night, these hormones' wires get crossed, leading to all kinds of problems with appetite, cravings, and portion control. If you never give your body a break from digesting, you don't make proper ghrelin, so you don't get proper hunger signals. If you never eat a hearty meal, you don't make proper leptin, so you don't experience proper fullness, also called satiety. Many people with type 2 and prediabetes have a hard time knowing when to eat, how much to eat, or, especially, when to stop eating. It's these two hormones, which are often out of balance, to blame.

Ghrelin and leptin are very powerful. Have you ever found yourself halfway through a snack or a dessert, before really being aware of eating it? You're not really hungry *or* full? Have you ever eaten something you know isn't good for you or you don't really want to eat but felt like you couldn't stop? You never really felt satisfied?

That's not *you*. That's not a failure of willpower. That's the twin gremlins: ghrelin and leptin, alongside some other chemicals (neurotransmitters) associated with reward and pleasure in the brain. These hormones are powerful. It helps to keep them in check. You *should* feel hungry in the morning, and before meals. At other times, you *shouldn't*. That's how the natural rhythm works.

This was the big win for Maria, as you may recall. Maria always felt so *hungry*. It was because she snacked all day and ate late at night. When she set this all to rights and began eating actual meals at appropriate times, her natural hunger signaling got back on track. She regained proper appetite. She restored feelings of sanity around how much to eat and when. All the natural goodness came flooding back.

Eat meals early in the day, and you can restore energy and freedom around food. You can get back in control if you've ever felt out of it. Restoring proper signaling by leptin and ghrelin can give you peace if you've ever felt stressed, guilty, confused, or ashamed of how much and when you're eating. It's not your fault. Give yourself the gift of meal timing.

TYING THE RHYTHM TOGETHER: OTHER INFLUENCES ON GHRELIN AND LEPTIN

If you can't tell when you're hungry, and you're eating the right portions at the right times, you may have to do some work with nutrition. The gut's microbiome influences ghrelin. If the microbiome is unhealthy—if you have too much of the bad gut bacteria and not enough of the good—your body might not make the right amount of ghrelin at the appropriate times.

Fiber and complex carbs/resistant starches help feed the gut's microbiome. Resistant starch is particularly helpful. You may also wish to include fermented foods like sauerkraut or kimchi in your diet to help feed good gut bacteria.

If you're eating the right portions at the right times, and you don't feel satisfied after meals, another reason could be poor sleep and/or chronic stress. Leptin relies on good sleep. If you need to snack a lot or feel like you can't stop eating, the root cause could be poor sleep. If you have sleep apnea or another sleep disorder, you may be especially vulnerable to this. Leptin also gets out of whack if your stress system is on overdrive. The more stressed you are, the less able your body is to send and receive leptin signals.

Remember: Progress, not perfection.

Reverend Lorraine

"The greatest gift for me was learning about the timing of meals. When I am consistent with the timing of my meals, and when I don't snack, that's the greatest gift. The challenge was always with not snacking: Two or three o'clock rolled around and I was the snack queen. But having the knowledge of meal timing and beginning to practice, to use Dr. Yates's language, has been the greatest gift."

THE IMPORTANCE OF RESETTING: WHY YOU SHOULDN'T SNACK

If you snack all day or regularly eat five or six mini meals, you can see your blood sugar rising up and up. It never has a chance to reset between meals.

The natural way your body maintains healthy blood sugar is by resetting between meals. You eat a meal, then you digest it. Your blood sugar goes up when eating, and your metabolic machinery works over the next hour or two to bring it back down. A few hours after that, you start to get hungry, and you can go ahead and prepare for your next meal. Your body is ready for it.

Chronically high blood sugar levels are toxic. It's imperative to bring them back down. The goal of reversing type 2 and prediabetes is to keep resetting lower and lower over time.

Snacking causes you to miss your opportunity for your blood sugar to reset.

Let's say your fasting morning number is 120. This is not ideal, but it's realistic for a lot of people with diabetes. When you eat breakfast, a good rise is about 30 points, but for someone with diabetes who's not yet on the Yates Protocol, it's likely going to be a bigger rise, maybe about 60 points. Okay. Now you're at 180. Two hours later, you decide to have a snack. But you haven't given your blood sugar enough time to come back down to 120, where it started. Let's say it's come halfway down, to 150. With the snack, it rises some more to 170. Then it's only another 3 hours until lunch. It won't fall back down to 120 in this time, either. Maybe it comes down to 150. You add 60 points again, just as you did with breakfast. Now you're up to 210. Then 2 hours later, you have a snack, but again it hasn't come back down all the way. You're stuck around 200. Dinner looms. Maybe you snack before and after.

Your blood sugar is really out of range, and all day it's kept inching higher and higher. It's been a slow but steady upward trend. This is trouble.

You might go to bed with your blood sugar over 200. Your body scrambles to digest all the food in your stomach and reset blood sugar overnight. But you've given it too much work. It can't reset well.

To heal type 2 and prediabetes, you must bring your numbers progressively lower. You can help your body do this through implementing healthy habits across all the steps of the Yates Protocol, but snacking can be a major obstacle that throws all the benefits of the program out the window.

Here's what happens when you eat in 3 meals.

Let's say your fasting morning number again is 120. You have breakfast. Ideally, it rises no more than 30 points, but to stay consistent, let's say it's 60 again. You're up to 180. This time you wait a full 5 hours until lunch, so you've reset back down to 120. You have lunch and it rises another 60 points, but you're up only to 180. You wait another 5 hours, and it falls back down before dinner. And here it rises again, too, but then you give yourself 3–5 hours before bedtime, so you're back down to 120 by the time you go to sleep. Since your blood sugar already has had time to reset down to this level, your body can bring it down even lower overnight. You might wake up the next day at 100 or 110. This is a big win. It's exactly what we want to see: resetting lower and lower over time. Progress isn't perfection, but the trend is what you want to see. Give yourself some grace, since healing isn't linear.

Over time, if you keep this up, and if you focus on eating healthy foods, meal timing, reducing stress, improving sleep, and exercising, you see these resets go down and down. Ideally, eventually, it will reset to the ideal morning blood sugar level of between 75 and 95.

PRO TIP: ASK YOURSELF WHY, LIKE REVEREND LORRAINE

My patient Reverend Lorraine always ate well, even before working with me. She cooked at home. She focused on whole and natural ingredients. But her meal timing was all off. The major problem was she was a snacker. Every afternoon she'd go have a snack. She loved the savory snacks: pretzels, cheese and crackers, a slice of toast with peanut butter. She was eating the whole-grain versions, but they were still carb heavy. When I told her about meal timing and the benefit of blood sugar resets, she understood immediately and decided to stop snacking for good. Whenever she found herself walking to the kitchen or break room at her church, she'd pause and ask herself why.

She knew that habits can be very powerful. So she didn't beat herself up. She just caught herself and asked if she was genuinely hungry. If she was, she'd have a little bit of a high-fat or protein snack, then commit to eating more food at lunch the next day. If she wasn't hungry, she would just stay busy.

We can get into habits, but we can always get out of them. Be present and intentional with yourself, with grace. Remember: Progress, not perfection.

SNACKING: DON'T, BUT IF YOU DO...

I don't recommend snacking. Full stop. I don't have any snack recipes. I don't promote snacking. I won't support it. If you're type 1, yes, snack as needed to avoid life-threatening low blood-sugar levels (hypoglycemia). Otherwise, no, don't snack.

Many of you will go ahead and snack anyway. If you are type 1 or are on a medication that requires snacking, that's a different story. But for most, once you meet your physiological needs and your leptin and ghrelin balance are in place, snacking is purely psychological. That's okay. It's okay to have psychological needs around food. Just understand that is why you're doing it. It's not a nutritional need.

Here are the snack guidelines I suggest so you don't completely lose the benefits of this blood-sugar healing journey.

You have two options. First, your snack is low fuel, aka low calorie. Make it vegetables, preferably raw, definitely *not* fried or baked in oil. If you like chips and crunchy things, replace them with slices of cucumber, with the skin on. Celery and radishes are similarly fibrous and very low fuel options. Carrots have more carbohydrate in them, so be careful and watch your blood sugar. You can add seasonings you enjoy.

The other option, which may be good for you if your blood sugar drops low, is higher fuel but still low carb: a small snack of protein with fats, possibly some fiber added. One option is to have a small portion of your favorite animal protein, such as one hard-boiled egg, or a small piece of meat. You could add some tomato salsa. Add some fiber if you like, a small amount, perhaps some raw or steamed broccoli or celery. Another option is high fat: You could have half a handful of nuts or seeds, or some nut or seed butter on a stick of celery (not a piece of fruit), but no more than a tablespoon.

I need to call out a common and dangerous myth: energy bars. They are bad snacks. They are usually mishmashes of sugar and other appetite stimulating chemicals, with some kind of highly processed carb or protein source thrown in the mix. They might advertise "high protein!" on the packaging, but check the label. If it's not at least 20 grams of protein, ditch it. If it's full of ingredients you don't recognize, ditch it. Look out for sources of carbohydrates, sugar, and fake sugar. Oats, barley, grain—these are supposedly "great fuel sources," but they're typically refined into simple carbs. Some energy bars are all "natural" but still high in sugar: Dried fruits are processed and especially high in sugar. Make decisions about what to eat that supports your healing, appetite, and blood sugar.

INTERMITTENT FASTING: TIMED WINDOWS FOR HEALING

Bee first contacted me on the cusp of her fiftieth birthday.

"Dr. Yates, am I supposed to develop insulin resistance and prediabetes in menopause?"

Inwardly, I sighed. Of course not. *But it does happen sometimes due to a combination of various sources of metabolic damage and the hormone changes women go through during this period. Sometimes, women are even told "This is normal, just accept it."*

Bee told me she had been going through menopause for a few years. She'd been dealing as best she could with some of the more typical symptoms like hot flashes. She didn't love those, but she could deal with them. What was driving her nuts was her rising blood sugar numbers. First, she began slowly developing insulin resistance. Then she was diagnosed with prediabetes. Her A1C was 5.8 percent.

Her doctor said it was normal: "It's natural when your progesterone drops that you lose some insulin sensitivity." About her prediabetic status, he added: "You're not diabetic technically, it's just prediabetes, so you don't have to do anything yet."

As Bee related this to me, I felt my heart sink. But I was also filled with relief that she had found me. We could find a way forward together.

As Bee and I talked more, I learned that she was already very health-conscious and most of her behaviors were in pretty good alignment with the Yates Protocol. We made sure her meals were composed of the 50 percent high-fiber vegetables, 25 percent lean protein, and 25 percent complex carbs/resistant starch. We added morning weight-lifting 3 times a week to her routine.

Then we gave her one extra boost: We added intermittent fasting.

Bee began eating all her meals within an 8-hour window between 10 a.m. and 6 p.m. From 6 p.m. until 10 a.m the next day, she did not eat. She had only unsweetened beverages: water, tea, or plain coffee.

Three months after that, Bee was able to email her previous doctor to inform him that both her A1C and fasting insulin levels had dropped into the middle of the healthy range.

AMPLIFYING THE HEALING BENEFITS OF THE BASIC RHYTHM WITH INTERMITTENT FASTING

The basic meal timing rhythm that I most often start patients on is 3 meals a day, spaced 4–5 hours apart, concluding 3–5 hours before bedtime. This is a great, healthy rhythm that gives your body at least 12 hours to reset blood sugar overnight.

But you can make one change to this rhythm with intermittent fasting (IF): Delay or skip breakfast and have a bigger lunch. This expands the amount of time you spend fasting overnight, from 12 hours to 14, 16, or 18 hours. That extra time can be a great gift.

There are many styles of IF (read more about them in the Resources section on the website), but the one I recommend most is this simple expansion of the time you spend fasting overnight.

Sometimes people call IF a Timed Window for Eating, or Time-Restricted Eating. Because IF can be so beneficial, I like to call it a Timed Window for *Healing*.

IF is my favorite way to help patients with type 2 and prediabetes quickly and safely achieve a better level of health, reduce cravings, lower A1C and fasting blood-sugar levels, and lose weight, if needed. IF improves cholesterol, insulin sensitivity, and an important kind of cellular repair the immune system carries out, called autophagy. It improves the quality of hormone signaling and can even help with the circadian rhythm.

Humans have been fasting for spiritual and health reasons for thousands of years. It's a natural practice that many of us have long forgotten. In the last ten years or so, many doctors and experts have begun recommending IF to help with all sorts of health issues, especially blood sugar, insulin, and excess weight. The wisdom is being rediscovered and reclaimed.

HOW TO INTERMITTENTLY FAST

The ideal tactic is 18 hours of fasting followed by a 6-hour eating window. If this 18:6 pattern works well for you, try this routine: Skip breakfast. Eat lunch at noon, and dinner at 6 p.m. Fast from 6 p.m. until noon the next day. Make sure your lunch is hearty. Do not snack.

You can also try a 16:8 pattern, with an 8-hour eating window from 10 a.m. to 6 p.m. Or an 8 a.m. to 6 p.m. eating window, which is a nice and gentle 14:10 pattern. That's a great option for anyone who wants to ease into IF.

Do not consume any food during this fasting window. Do not consume any flavored beverages, though unsweetened coffee and tea might be okay.

You can progressively increase your fasting period overnight if it feels good for you: first thirteen, then fourteen, then fifteen hours, etc.

Just delay breakfast a bit more, slowly over time. It's important to be realistic with all the steps and focus on sustainable change.

Even when intermittently fasting, always eat proper meals. IF is not an invitation to snack. If your eating window is still on the larger end, for example 12 or 10 hours, you might still have three meals. You can have a delayed breakfast, then wait 4 hours before lunch and 4 before dinner. Alternatively, you can turn this into a two-meal situation with a big break between meals. In that case, still allocate most of your calories to your first meal.

It's best not to fuss too much about calories and trying to make sure you eat any precise amount. Wait 15 minutes after eating to see if you still feel hungry. If you find yourself eating very fast or a lot more than normal, or your hunger signals start to feel off, revert to three meals in the same window or a bigger eating window. If you feel yourself getting "hangry" or starting to obsess over food, relax the strategy and maybe revisit it another time.

Keep an eye out for any potential issues cropping up. For many, IF improves a wide variety of symptoms. But for others, IF can spell too much stress. For women especially, this could lead to skin, thyroid, and hormone issues. Watch out for skin quality, potential changes to your menstrual cycle (many see improvements, but not all), or other reproductive hormone changes. Make sure your sleep and stress improve, not worsen.

KEEP HEALTHY MEALS

Some influencers say you can snack throughout your whole eating window. For example: Johnny Influencer says *Eat freely in your eight-hour eating window.*

Some others say you can eat whatever you want. Susie Influencer says *Eat whatever you like! Go ahead and eat highly processed, ultra-refined food!*

These are dangerous myths.

Do not snack. Two or three meals a day is the rule, no matter if you're intermittent fasting or not. You still want your blood sugar to reset between meals.

Eating is an opportunity to repair metabolic damage with healthy foods. No matter how good IF or anything is for you, if you don't hit the nutritional bull's-eye at the center of health and build your body out of the right stuff, with the right timing, you're wasting a huge opportunity and possibly preventing your ability to heal.

PRO TIP: FEAST WITH HEALTHY MEALS, LIKE ALAN

Alan first got in touch with me after attending one of my online seminars. He told me he was confused because he had been intermittently fasting with a 6-hour eating window (an 18:6 pattern) for several weeks and not seeing any of the benefits he had been hoping for. He wasn't losing weight, but even more importantly, his A1C wasn't going down. When he'd started, it was 8.0 percent, and it had come down only to 7.8 percent.

I asked Alan about his nutrition. He had seen on social media that you could eat basically whatever you felt like when doing IF. Alan had a ritual: After a long workday, he'd have pizza, followed by dessert. He'd thought IF would "make up" for these choices.

When I explained to Alan that IF was a way to amplify the benefits of healthy eating, *not replace healthy eating*, he understood right away.

Now he was going to have a dinner that nourished both his spirit *and* his body: grass-fed beefburgers with sweet potato buns, homemade greens he'd prepared ahead of time, artisanal salad dressing made with organic, cold-pressed, extra-virgin olive oil. Alan began giving himself the gift of looking forward to a nice feast for dinner, but this time a real *feast* full of nourishing and delicious foods.

Alan began to see progress in his fasting morning blood sugars and A1C after that. He also noticed that he stopped getting "hangry" the following morning, too.

INTERMITTENT FASTING IS NOT FOR EVERYBODY

Pregnant and breastfeeding women should not practice IF.

Children and adolescents are growing. Do not IF!

Some people who have histories of yo-yo dieting or unhealthy emotional relationships with food find that they regain some amount of freedom with IF—but many are the opposite. If the idea of IF makes you uncomfortable or you start experimenting with it and feel like old habits with eating disorders are coming back into place, stop. It's not for you. Psychological health is a priority. You can't eat well if you're not in the right headspace for it. Prioritize what you must to heal your relationship with food. IF can play a role in your health journey later, or never. Being at peace with food is important.

TEST, DON'T GUESS

If you decide to implement IF, watch your blood sugar numbers. How are your readings after meals and when you wake up the next morning? Are you resetting lower? That's what you want to see. Don't obsess about any one data point, but over the course of weeks you should be able to see general trends. Keep tweaking to find the eating rhythm that works best for you, and consider it alongside proper nutrition, exercise, sleep, and stress management strategies.

SWITCH IT UP

Whatever you do, it must be sustainable. If daily IF doesn't work well for you, you could try creating a different schedule, such as fasting on alternate days or weeks.

It's important to be consistent, but such alternating patterns *are* consistent. For example, research has shown that a fasting mimicking diet (FMD)—fasting with food (very specific, researched ingredients) for 5 days a month, for between 3 and 12 months—can produce profound effects. It's got variation in it, but it's from a three-month to a twelve-month cycle. The body learns to switch between fat-burning and fuel-storage modes. (Research has validated this, and people's experiences affirm it.) You can find out more in the Resources section of the website.

You could implement IF every other day, or only weekdays, only weekends, one week a month. Consistency matters, so once you find the eating window that works for you, switch only between that and your baseline. When in a fasting week, eat your fasting schedule. When in a baseline week, eat your baseline.

In this chapter, you learned:

- The basic rhythm that supports health: 3 meals a day, spaced 4–5 hours apart, concluding 3–5 hours before bedtime.

- The biggest mistake most people make is skipping lunch, leading to increased appetite, becoming "hangry," and having more difficulty making healthy choices later. Lunch is self-care. Do not skip lunch.

- Always bring your own healthy meals. Preparedness is self-care.

- Snacking is a major obstacle to blood sugar health. Unless you are type 1, do not snack.

- Intermittent fasting is another eating rhythm that can accelerate blood sugar healing.

- If you are pregnant, breastfeeding, or a teenager or child, do not IF.

- If you begin IF and experience any symptoms, stop.

Quick wins/first steps:

- Get rid of snacks. Donate them, give them to neighbors, or throw them away.

- Have a hearty, savory breakfast rich in fiber and lean protein every day for a week. Test your blood sugar and see how you feel.

- Give yourself the gift of lunch for at least two weeks.

- Prepare a healthy lunch ahead of time.

- Eat filling meals. Fill your plate according to Yates Protocol portions. After eating, wait fifteen minutes. If still hungry, eat more.

CHAPTER 3

Sleep

These 3 Steps to Better Sleep Might Be What You
Need to Improve Your Blood Sugar and A1C Levels

CHAPTER MAP

This chapter explains the importance of long and
deep sleep; my 3-step road map offers tips in six
crucial domains.

KEY SECTIONS

- Night and day: the body's natural rhythm
- Stress and poor sleep: two silent, intertwined
  causes of type 2 and prediabetes
- A 3-step road map to long and deep sleep
- Implement six tips to help yourself sleep
- Two deadly circumstances that must be addressed:
  shift work and sleep apnea

Sonia blinked at me and rubbed her eyes.

"Sorry, what was that? I'm just really tired. I mean I'm used to being tired, but I'm just extra tired today."

How many patients have said similar things to me?

Sonia and I were having our first of many Zoom consultations. I asked again, "Tell me about your sleep situation."

"My biggest challenge," she told me, "is getting proper sleep. It's not that I don't want proper sleep, but I can't get it. I am a caregiver to my daughter. She's forty-seven and has a seizure disorder. She will often go nights without sleeping, and that keeps me up. So that's my biggest challenge."

I understood. Many of my patients were in difficult situations with sleep. Sonia went on to tell me more details that compounded the difficulty.

She sometimes sets alarms for the middle of the night to check on her daughter. Even when her daughter is deep asleep, Sonia can sleep fitfully because she's worried. Other times, Sonia will just lie in her own bed and think about everything she has to do the next day to keep the family afloat.

It is a lot to carry.

Sonia wasn't getting the long and deep rest she needed, and this was the core reason she was recently diagnosed with type 2.

Sonia's situation was difficult, not hopeless. First we reduced Sonia's exposure to the blue light from computer and TV screens. Then she started supplementing with magnesium and replaced her synthetic bed linens with cotton ones that would help prevent overheating. We also devised practical changes to her life. She became proactive about getting support (not just for her daughter, but for *herself*). Eventually, she started to get on the right track with nutrition, meal timing, and exercise, too.

When Sonia and I had first connected, her A1C was 7.5 percent and her fasting blood sugar (FBS) was 140 mg/dl. Anything 6.5 percent and above, or 126 and above, signals type 2 diabetes. Today her

A1C is 6.4 percent and her FBS is 100. This is *remission* and represents wonderful, steady progress.

Do you want to have better blood sugar and A1C levels? Go to sleep. Do you need help with your aches and pains, your stress, your mood, your energy? Go to sleep. Do you want to help weight loss efforts? Go to sleep.

Sleep matters.

But in many cases, going to sleep and staying asleep are more easily said than done.

SLEEP MATTERS

Quality sleep is as essential to survival as food and water. It is vital to blood sugar management and recovering from type 2 and prediabetes. For some people, it is the most essential of all the steps of the Yates Protocol. Sleep is the foundation of all health.

Sometimes, the number one factor driving poor blood-sugar numbers and insulin sensitivity is poor sleep.

Chronic sleep deprivation, even as few as five consecutive nights of short sleep, is associated with an increased risk of obesity, insulin resistance, and type 2 and prediabetes.

NO MATTER HOW HEALTHY YOUR LIFESTYLE, REDUCED SLEEP INCREASES RISK

In a 2023 study of a quarter million people in the UK, researchers determined that people who sleep fewer than six hours a night have a notably higher risk of type 2 than those who get seven to eight hours of sleep. This is even accounting for whether they eat healthfully. Independent of diet, people who sleep less are at greater risk of developing type 2.

Today, 20 percent of Americans get fewer than five hours of sleep a night. In 1942, that number was 3 percent. Between 1942 and today, our society has gone from 1 in 33 to 1 in 5 people suffering from this major risk.

OTHER RELATED HEALTH EFFECTS

Sleep affects every tissue and organ in the body. The body repairs muscles, grows tissues, and synthesizes proteins at night. It makes key immune molecules that fight infection and inflammation. It releases many critical hormones, including sex hormones.

Sleep is especially crucial for the brain. When you sleep, your brain solidifies the new information and memories you've experienced that day. If you don't sleep, you more easily forget what's happened or anything you've learned. Sleep flushes toxins out of the brain. It restructures and reorganizes nerve cells.

Sleep affects mood and resilience. If you're chronically irritable, have a short fuse, feel on edge all day, or feel like you can't handle as much as you'd like, poor sleep could be the reason. It's not your fault. The brain's centers for emotional regulation refresh while you sleep.

Serious chronic health problems related to poor sleep include obesity, weight gain, food cravings, memory disorders, dementia (aka type 3 diabetes), Alzheimer's (the most common subtype of dementia), mood disorders, immune system disorders, autoimmune disease, heart disease, and, of course, insulin resistance, prediabetes, and type 2 diabetes.

After a good night's sleep, you wake feeling refreshed. It's a direct outcome of the body doing all these important processes. If you don't feel refreshed when you wake, you are likely not getting long and deep enough sleep to restore health the way you need.

PRO TIP: MAKE "NOT REFRESHED" YOUR WAKE-UP CALL

In a recent Gallup poll, 57 percent of Americans said they'd feel better if they got more rest, compared to 42 percent who said they felt like they slept as much as they needed. This is about the opposite of ten years before, when 56 percent said they got the sleep they needed and 43 percent did not. Many aren't feeling refreshed, but they keep going anyway. This is a serious health risk. That "not refreshed" feeling is the tip of the iceberg. Beneath that can be a whole ocean of poor markers of health.

"Not refreshed" is a wake-up call for change.

NIGHT AND DAY: THE BODY'S NATURAL RHYTHM

In chapter 2, I introduced the concept of the body's natural rhythm and how it's tied to the rhythm of the earth. Sleep is a crucial element of this rhythm. As the sun rises, your body wants to wake up. When the sun is high in the sky, your body expects to be active, burning what you've eaten as fuel.

As the sun begins to set, your body wants to be winding down. It wants to get slow and sleepy, to rest and replenish. This is a natural rhythm, and every cell in your body works best when in harmony with it. Prioritize sleep, and you get on your body's side, letting it relax into the natural rhythm it was designed for. Much of the brokenness of our modern world comes from being out of sync with what's natural for us. Give yourself the gift of this ancient harmony.

HOW MUCH SLEEP TO GET

For most adults ages twenty-five to seventy, aim for 7.5 to 8 hours of sleep a night. Go to bed early enough to give yourself the opportunity to sleep that long. If it takes you some time to fall asleep, factor that in. With good sleep hygiene, you should be able to fall asleep quicker.

If you're older, your sleep window might shrink. As long as you wake up feeling refreshed and ready for your day, don't worry about only getting 6 hours. You can't really force that. If you don't feel refreshed, then you can work on this. Dial in your sleep hygiene to see if you can increase that window.

Teens need as much sleep as toddlers: 10 to 12 hours a day. If we were kinder to our teens, we'd start school later, so they'd have enough time to get the rest they need. Physiologically they aren't going to *want* to go to bed sooner: Teens typically undergo a physiological change where they naturally go to sleep and wake up on a later schedule. If you're a teen or there are teens in your life struggling with blood sugar management, do what you can to prioritize sleep and maintain healthy sleep hygiene.

LARKS AND OWLS

Some of us are naturally night owls and go to bed later. Some are morning larks. Most are somewhere in between. It's a spectrum. This is genetic. We all have *chronomeres* that incline us to rest earlier or later. Chronomeres are small, linear DNA molecules that are thought to be part of the chromosome structure.

One is not more virtuous or better than the other. In human history, larks and owls may have played different roles. Today, we often celebrate and accommodate larks. We praise the early bird getting the worm. Our world is designed for the lark schedule. It's relatively easy for larks to get up and go to work in the early morning hours, and to perform their best at these times. Owls are equally productive and energetic human beings—but with a different timing.

Owls can suffer as a result. If you're naturally a night owl, it's great if in your working years you have a job that has you start later. If you force yourself to get up for a job at 6, 7, or 8 a.m. but have a genetic inclination to go to sleep and wake later, you're burning both ends of the candle. This is a recipe for type 2 and prediabetes. One study suggests that night owls are at higher risk of prediabetes and type 2—but maybe only if forced to wake up before they're ready.

If you're naturally a night owl, be aware of this and do what you can to accommodate your needs. Get a job that makes sense for the demands of your body if you can. If not, experiment with sleep hygiene. See if you can switch to an earlier schedule even if it feels unnatural at first. Allocate at least 7.5 to 8 hours for rest.

HOW TO KNOW WHEN YOU REST BEST

How do you know if you're a lark or an owl, or somewhere in between?

When you have a quiet, calm evening with no surprises, not a lot of craziness going on, pay attention. When does your energy naturally drop? Notice that release of the "sleep hormone" melatonin as it seeps out from your pineal gland at night. You start to yawn. You move slower. Your eyelids start to feel heavy. Do this several times. See if the natural drop happens around the same time. It should!

It's ideal to do this after you've started implementing some of the sleep tips I recommend below, especially setting a screen curfew or installing orange light filters on your screens, as the bright, blue light at night disrupts your circadian rhythm.

I naturally get tired quite predictably around 9:00 p.m. I give myself about 90 minutes to wind down and move toward bed. Then I make it a point to be in bed no later than 10:45 p.m. How long do you like or need to wind down? What bedtime enables you to rest long and deep? Find a routine that works for you.

CONSISTENCY IS KEY

The body gets used to rhythms. Sleep and wake around the same time every day, with up to about an hour of variance.

Don't make big changes across the days of the week, weekend, or vacations or holidays. If you usually go to bed at 11:00 p.m., that's fine. Plan on 8 hours of sleep: Wake at 7:00 a.m. But you don't then want to go to bed at 1:00 a.m. or 2:00 a.m. on the weekends, or to get up at 10:30 or 11:00 a.m. That's too big a difference from your normal schedule. You can flex your bedtime by around an hour, but the more consistent you are, the better. Your body will reward you with better overall hormonal balance, including insulin production being more consistent.

So many of us are so used to this hustle culture of pushing through. If you're tired at night, don't push through. Sometimes you get a "second wind," but that's not a good thing. You're forcing your body to stay awake when it wants to rest and repair. You're chipping into your natural sleeping window. You can't get that sleep back. Even if you sleep in, the quality of sleep you get will likely be diminished because your cells are off schedule.

I recently wanted to finish some extra work before sleep. It was 8:30 p.m. I needed at least two hours to get the work done. I *technically* could have completed the task before my 10:45 p.m. sleep time, but I knew that working hard until 10:30 p.m. wouldn't leave enough time to wind down properly. I'd never be ready and relaxed enough by my normal 10:45 p.m. I had to ask myself: What kind of life do I want to live? Do I want to cave to the demands of hustle culture and push through, or do I want to set boundaries against it? Do I want to prioritize my health? Do I want to be that change for myself and others?

I decided I would do the work the next day. Fortunately, this was an option available to me. I need to listen to my body: *What is my body telling me?* Sometimes I absolutely must stay up later than my body wants. Okay. But if I can—and if I'm honest with myself, I almost always can—I prioritize sleep.

NAPPING AND "CATCHING UP": DON'T DO IT

Napping, in general, and on occasion is okay. It won't hurt your health! But it shouldn't be relied upon in place of a good night's rest. Sleep is best when long and deep at night. This is when restoration and blood sugar resetting happen.

Some cultures, many in warmer parts of the world, have naps built into the daily rhythm. It works for them. Why? They're still getting good sleep overnight! They also have less stress. A slower pace of life interacts with the body clock differently. Humans are always very context dependent. What works for one person or group of people in one context may not in another.

Generally, in today's world and looking at the data we have on sleep, it seems to be better for overall sleep quality and wellness if you go through your day without a nap.

Long naps can reduce sleep quality at night. When you wake up in the morning, and especially if you get early morning sun exposure, your body sets a 14-hour timer for when it will begin to make melatonin and put you to sleep that night. But you also need something called *sleep pressure* to build throughout the day. Your body creates sleep pressure by producing *adenosine*. Adenosine levels rise while awake throughout the day. (Bonus: You make more if you exercise.) When you sleep, napping included, your body clears out the adenosine. Napping reduces the amount of sleep pressure for nighttime.

Stay curious about your blood sugar numbers and sleep quality. If you're finding that your quality of life and health are better with a nap, do it. If you're finding a nap means you want to go to bed later or you're not getting the same amount of sleep, you might want to let that nap go.

If your sleep is at a deficit and you're dragging during the day, care for yourself. A nap might feel good and help restore mental clarity and energy. Fifteen or thirty minutes earlier in the day, before 2 p.m., may work well. You likely won't derail your mounting sleep pressure.

Don't cheat yourself on sleep at night with the intent to make up for it with a nap. The truth is: You can't catch up on sleep. Once it's gone, it's gone! Many say, *Oh, I'll just take a nap.* It's not the same. If you've missed a night's sleep, it is not coming back.

A similar thing happens with the weekends. Some people sleep five or six hours a night during the week, then say they'll catch up on the weekend. This is a terrible pattern. Science does not support this. It leads to much higher risk of metabolic damage, including elevated blood sugar and A1C and struggles with weight. Care for yourself, please. Be honest with yourself.

SETTING UP YOUR NIGHT WITH YOUR DAY: LIGHT

To reset to lower blood sugar levels overnight and awaken with happy morning blood sugar numbers, you'll need the day before to make sense. Daytime success sets up nighttime success.

One crucial element of a successful day is light. Light is the most important source of information cells use to set their circadian rhythm clocks. Today's world has really messed up our relationship with light. If you want proper light exposure, you must go out and get it. You must make an effort.

As soon as possible after waking up, go outside and get at least 15 minutes of direct natural light. Get the sun on your skin if possible. Walk if possible. If there's inclement weather, try sitting on a porch or by a window. Even for blind people, it makes a difference. The light comes through your eyelids and is received by your retina. It's also received by your skin cells.

When the bright light of the sun first streams into your eyes and skin, and the signal hits your brain, you stop making the sleep hormone melatonin and set an internal timer to start making it again about 14 hours later. This creates a critical anchor for your body's circadian rhythm. Regular morning light can be as powerful or more powerful than a cup of coffee, exercise, or an alarm for helping entrain your circadian rhythm.

In the winter, don't change this routine. If the days get dark and cloudy, you can purchase a sun lamp and look toward it for at least 15 minutes. It's not as good as the natural sun, but it can deliver a helpful boost. Some people use alarm clocks that double as lamps and gradually increase light to mimic the rise of the sun.

As you go about your day, keep exposing yourself to bright, hopefully natural, light. Abundant studies demonstrate the power of natural light exposure: Regular time in natural light, whether through your windows or spending time outside, is associated with faster, deeper sleeping and improved mood and health. One study found that when people let natural light stream into their apartments for one week, they fell asleep 22 minutes earlier, slept more regularly, and reported an overall more positive affect than those without light streaming in.

As the day draws to a close, continue to mimic the natural conditions as best you can by turning off the lights. Bright lights stimulate wakefulness. That includes the light from your TV, computer, laptop, and phone screens.

Screens can be especially problematic because their default setting is to emit blue light, which is the frequency of light that most stimulates wakefulness. This is different from the light of the sun, which is white.

Using screens at night can significantly delay sleep onset and disrupt your circadian rhythm.

Fortunately, many phones, tablets, and laptops now have the option to program night modes that change the frequency of the light on your screen from blue to orange. Think of the orange light of the sunset or a campfire. It doesn't stimulate wakefulness the same way the blue light of screens does. Turn your night/orange filters on. If you don't have orange light functionality built into your devices, you can download apps that do it, or overlay a screen that blocks blue light. Some devices also have "dark mode" options where some of the software on them runs with a black background.

It's best to set a curfew on screens entirely, such as by 90 minutes before bed. Before that, it is okay to use the screens in orange or dark mode. Experiment for yourself and find what works for you.

Take stock of the kinds of light bulbs you have in your home. Different bulbs emit different frequency light. You may wish to swap out bluer, cool tone bulbs or pure white bulbs for warmer, orange tinted ones. You can purchase LED lights at specific frequencies. Orange or other warm-colored shades can help. Some companies manufacture blue-light-blocking glasses. Many people who are sensitive to blue light benefit from them 90 minutes or more before bed. Dim lighting is always best at night. You may even wish to try switching to candlelight after the sun sets.

SETTING UP THE NIGHT WITH THE DAY: THE OTHER STEPS

The other four steps of the Yates Protocol—nutrition, meal timing, exercise, and stress—all impact sleep.

Nutrition

Your body needs sufficient nutrients to sleep well. Make sure you get sufficient protein, fat, and complex carbohydrate/resistant starch in each meal. All of them nourish the brain and support the production of various hormones and neurotransmitters necessary for sleep. Pay special attention to vegetables, especially leafy greens, nourishing fats from grass-fed, pasture-raised, wild-caught animal products, and nourishing fats from avocados, seeds, nuts, and coconuts, as they contain crucial vitamins and minerals that can help you make the hormones you need for long and deep sleep.

Meal timing

Eating out of sync with your natural rhythm is a major source of clock confusion. The body expects to get most of its nutrients earlier in the day. If you delay this, you may end up confusing your clock, leading to difficulty falling asleep, waking in the middle of the night, or disrupted sleep. Earlier meals are typically better for regulating the circadian rhythm.

Exercise

Exercise, especially vigorous exercise, causes the body to produce cortisol, the body's main wakefulness and stress hormone. Cortisol's main job is to keep you awake. Cortisol levels need to be lower at night for your circadian rhythm to be on track.

For many people with prediabetes and type 2 diabetes, the best time to exercise is before breakfast. Exercise in a fasted state right when you wake up, and you help bring your blood sugar down as well as give your body a wakefulness boost that kicks off the circadian rhythm. Going for a run or walk outside and it's a two-fer: You get both exercise and natural sunlight at the same time.

If fasted early-morning exercise doesn't work for you, exercise at some point in the morning or afternoon: after breakfast or during your lunch break.

Finish your exercise, especially if strenuous, 5 hours before bed. As the sun begins to set, the body naturally wants to move more slowly and start shutting down. This doesn't mean you have to give up doing activities at night, but pay attention. If your sleep is not good, if you don't feel rested, or if your morning blood sugar is high, this is an area to give more attention.

Stress management

Finally, stress causes the body to produce excessive cortisol. If you are chronically stressed or if you do things that stress you late in the day (having stressful conversations, working late, being on email at all hours), this can throw off your rhythm. Stress can seem overwhelming and impossible to reduce or manage, but it can be done. Make it a priority. It really matters. I describe the health effects of stress and how to manage it in chapter 5.

STRESS AND POOR SLEEP: TWO SILENT, INTERTWINED CAUSES OF TYPE 2 AND PREDIABETES

Meet Len.

The clock ticked over from 4:43 to 4:44 a.m. Len's eyes snapped open. He did a quick body scan. Heart rate elevated but not in a dangerous range. He heaved himself up and swung his legs over the edge of the bed. He had to get up, grab the bag on the floor by the door, shower and dress, and be out the door in twenty minutes. Okay. He reached over to his nightstand to switch off the alarm, and paused. He realized: The alarm never went off. It was 4:46 and the alarm hadn't gone off.

"Wait, Len, wait." Wait, he said to himself. "Len, there is no alarm! You're retired!"

As Len later told me, he then sighed and lay back down to stare at the ceiling. The thing is, Len was in the habit of getting up and going. His body was ready for it. It naturally anticipated an alarm that no longer rang.

Len had served in the military for thirty-one years, on call 24/7, and always had a bag packed, ready to deploy within forty-eight hours at a moment's notice. He told me that sleep—or any of his needs—had never been his priority.

"A lot of the aches and pains you ignore because you don't have time for it," he said.

Len had not woken up slowly in thirty-one years. He always woke at 4:45 a.m. sharp, no matter what time he made it to bed. "What a hard habit to break, Dr. Yates! I keep telling myself—chill out, man! You can sleep in! You don't have to keep running!"

Throughout Len's long military career, he had eaten as well as he was able. He had exercised. He had cared for his body to the best of his ability. But the truth is, his body got wired for stress, and he rarely prioritized sleep. He had loved his job and served his country with integrity and pride, but the kind of work he did kept his body in go *mode.*

Poor sleep may not have been the only cause of Len's type 2 diagnosis, but it played a role. When you combine it with the go go go, *constant alert* mode Len had been in for thirty-one years, *it is especially powerful. Stress and poor sleep often go hand in hand and can exacerbate the damaging effects.*

I had the joy and privilege of watching Len begin to unwind. It took some time. It usually does! But implementing tips like the ones I provide can help accelerate the process.

Today, Len still does a lot. He spends most of his waking time caring for his family and volunteering. But sleep is a priority. For him, one major aspect of his healing is just going back to sleep. He's going at a slower pace today and always prioritizing his sleep.

"What a gift sleep is, Dr. Yates!"

Americans are sleeping less than ever before. For the first time ever, more than half (57 percent) report failing to get the sleep they need. At the same time, more report stress in daily life: as of 2023, 49 percent. There is significant overlap between these groups. Of those who report wanting more sleep, 63 percent say they frequently experience stress.

Both poor sleep and stress cause type 2 and prediabetes on their own. Combined, they become a mutually escalating tornado of metabolic damage.

Poor sleep contributes to feelings of stress by degrading the mental and physical resources for coping with the trials of life. It can make you feel weary or hypervigilant. When you don't rest long and deep, your brain does not have the opportunity it needs to refresh. Sleep is the greatest opportunity to repair the metabolic damage caused by stress. Sacrifice sleep and you suffer more from stress.

Stress contributes to poor sleep by putting the body in fight-or-flight mode. Stress can cause you to stay awake staring at the ceiling, too wound up to fall asleep, to wake in the middle of the night in a jolt of panic, or to wake earlier than ideal. You lose that precious time for repair and blood sugar resetting. You become less resilient to stress the next day. It is a vicious cycle.

One common outcome of simultaneous poor sleep and stress is haywire appetite. The appetite hormones ghrelin and leptin are highly sensitive to both poor sleep and stress. Many stressed and under-slept people don't feel hungry or full when they would otherwise, leading to snacking, runaway cravings, and that dangerous late-night eating. If this is you, it's not your fault. Poor sleep and stress are powerful intertwined forces on the trajectory into metabolic damage.

Today, there is a great deal of alarm being raised over the rising rates of obesity and its potential links with type 2. But I wonder: What about potential links between rising rates of poor sleep and stress and type 2 and prediabetes?

This is a potential link we must give more attention to. It is literally a matter of life and death.

The growing danger of mixed poor sleep and stress appears to be greatest for women, and especially young women. In 2023, 53 percent of women, compared to 45 percent of men, reported frequent stress. Women between ages eighteen and forty-nine are the most likely of all groups to express frequent stress, exceeding men in their age group by 14 points. In this age group, 69 percent of women (55 percent of men) report frequent stress. Younger women are the least likely to report getting adequate sleep, at only 27 percent (compared to 46 percent of men in this age group).

Take stock of your life and be honest with yourself. How much stress and burden do you carry for yourself and for others? Is your stress disproportionate? What steps can you take to change this?

SLEEP AND THE GREMLINS OF APPETITE:
IT'S NOT YOUR FAULT

Sleep has a profound effect on the twin gremlins leptin and ghrelin (page 52). During sleep, ghrelin, which stimulates appetite, naturally decreases. Leptin, which suppresses appetite, naturally increases. Lack of sleep disrupts this natural balance. Ghrelin goes *up* and leptin goes *down*. You get the opposite of what you want. You get more of the hormone that says, "*I'm hungry!*" and less of the hormone that says, "*I'm full!*" This can make it harder to tell when it's time to stop eating and can lead to struggles with overeating.

The day after a night of poor sleep, you will be much more likely to feel hungry, to snack, to eat bigger meals than normal, and to eat junk. Your blood sugar regulation will likely also be worse because of the poor sleep, making this a dangerous duo.

If you chronically under-sleep, this can be real trouble. Feelings of being hungry or "hangry" can become the new normal for you. You can end up feeling like you could always eat more, no matter how much you eat. It can become harder and harder to keep your meals the size your body needs. It's not your fault. These hormones are very powerful. Prioritize sleep and you make it easier to nourish yourself well with the right foods and to eat them in the right amounts at the right times.

THE DAWN PHENOMENON: WAKING UP WITH
ELEVATED BLOOD SUGAR

All people get a natural bump of cortisol in the early morning hours. This is your system starting to kick online. For most people, cortisol starts streaming gently into the bloodstream around 4 or 5 a.m., with a wake time around 7 a.m. The time varies according to your circadian rhythm, sleep habits, and genetics.

Every time cortisol goes up, blood sugar goes up with it. It's a part of how the body prepares itself for action. For a healthy person without blood sugar issues, the rise in blood sugar at this time is just a few points. No biggie. For some with type 2 and prediabetes, it's greater than that. For about half of people with type 2 or prediabetes, it's *significantly* greater: 40, 50, 100 points. This is too much.

This is known as an exaggerated dawn phenomenon.

Test your blood sugar in the morning immediately upon waking. Is it elevated, even if you rested long and deep? Do this several days in a row. Does it continue to be elevated? You may be experiencing the dawn phenomenon.

If you are, it's especially important to have good sleep hygiene. The last few hours of sleep—whether they occur for you in the typical 4 to 7 a.m. range or slightly later due to genetics—are important for the overall quality of sleep you get. If your body is shooting your blood sugar up by 40, 50, or 100 points before you are supposed to wake up, this is disruptive. You may start tossing and turning or wake up earlier than is ideal. Identify and implement the sleep techniques I describe later in this chapter to help you.

An exaggerated dawn phenomenon starts your day on a difficult foot. You want to begin with the lowest blood-sugar numbers possible in the healthy range, ideally the lowest that you experience in a 24-hour period. Then, as you go through your day and do things like eat meals, move around, exercise, and experience stress, your numbers rise but then fall back down and reset again overnight. If you start the day with numbers already elevated, you'll struggle to reset in a way that heals.

If you experience an exaggerated dawn phenomenon, it is important to avoid snacking, to exercise, and to keep moving throughout the day. This will help your blood sugar reset to lower levels between meals.

One thing you can do to reduce any harmful effects is to exercise: Before breakfast in a fasted state is best, if possible. This can help burn some of the excess blood sugar and give you a better starting point for your day. Some people prefer to exercise after breakfast. If that's your preference, that can work for you. But if you haven't yet tried exercising while in a fasted state, give it a shot. Monitor your numbers and how you feel. Just ten minutes of movement can make a difference and helps you start your day with a good baseline.

A 3-STEP ROAD MAP TO LONG AND DEEP SLEEP

1: Ask yourself: Are you willing to prioritize sleep?

First: Get your priorities right. Ask yourself: Am I willing to prioritize myself and my sleep? Am I giving myself enough time to sleep 7.5 to 8 hours a night? Am I respecting my needs for fun and relaxation? Am I taking time to wind down before bed? Take a moment to be honest with yourself.

If you go to bed at midnight and you know you have to get up at 6:30 a.m., you didn't give yourself enough hours. Sleep is a precious opportunity to hit that reset button on your blood sugar. You get another swing at the bat 24 hours later, but you can do only so much. You can't make up for missed sleep. You're digging a hole.

Some people naturally sleep 4 hours and feel fine. They are outliers. If you're sleeping 4, 5, 6 hours a night and feel great *and have great health and blood sugar levels*, good for you. But for the vast majority, that will not be the case. Pay attention and be honest with yourself. Get a wearable health monitoring device if you can and heed what it tells you about your sleep quality and needs. If you don't feel well rested in the morning, make changes.

If you wake up groggy, have sand in your eyes, and you're dragging your feet, if you need coffee to function, feel exhausted later in the day . . . if you have low energy, low mood, if you crash in the afternoon . . . you're probably not getting adequate sleep.

2: Identify: What triggers poor sleep?

It can take some time to identify your obstacles to sleep, but there are answers. Here is a list of some of the most common obstacles, though it is not exhaustive.

Alcohol. Alcohol has a sedative effect on the brain. This can help you fall asleep. But it also triggers detoxification processes that stimulate wakefulness, disrupting sleep. When you drink alcohol, you have lighter sleep, wake earlier, and increase the risk of sleep disruptions like hot flashes or needing to get up to urinate. This is one of the many reasons I recommend against regular alcohol consumption. Ideally, if you consume it, it's 5 hours or more before bed.

Screens before bed. Screens are bright, which stimulates wakefulness, and are typically blue tinted, which stimulates it even more. The blue light of screens can delay the onset of sleep by hours or prevent it entirely. Utilize orange light filters on screens after the sun sets and set a curfew for screens for at least 90 minutes before bed.

Trying to fall asleep with the TV, radio, or lights on. Some people distract themselves from racing thoughts or negative emotions by leaving some kind of programming running while they try to sleep. This can hurt sleep in the long run. You don't have to look right at a screen or light source for it to disrupt your body's rhythm. Skin cells can detect light, and your ears and brain are taking in that noise.

Violent or distressing content. Any movies, shows, or news feeds that have violent or distressing content can leave your mind and body buzzing. Be mindful of how you're mentally and emotionally setting winding down at the end of the day.

Social media. Social media can ensnare attention, often in negative ways, leading to a racing heart or mind. Don't fall down rabbit holes, especially if they're feeding fear or anger. Set boundaries for yourself around social media. Put it away at night if there's a chance it'll trigger negative feelings.

Stress. Your body and mind are deeply intertwined: Your body can't relax if your mind is ruminating. Intentionally relax your mind. Meditate. Pray. Take a bath. Journal. Read. Eliminate, manage, or reduce sources of stress in your life.

Doing "one more thing." Many people just go go go, right up until bed. Some lie down, remember something they had intended to do earlier, then get up and do it. They can end up like a jack-in-the-box, up and down and up and down. Some wake up in the middle of the night and perform tasks they forgot. Bed is a time for rest. Even if you can't sleep, give yourself the gift of rest. If you have an idea about something that needs to be done, write it down and revisit it later. You will be able to sort things on your to-do list when the sun is up, and your body and mind are more naturally equipped to tackle them.

3: Implement my six tips

There's a lot you can do to help yourself sleep. Read through this list and consider which changes may be most beneficial for you. Some are relatively low-hanging fruit. Using an eye mask or wearing ear plugs are both super cost-effective and simple changes that could make a big difference. Others may take some more work. Doing all of these is of course ideal, but make change at a pace that is right for you.

Sleep timing

GO TO BED AT THE SAME TIME EACH NIGHT.
You can vary bedtime by up to an hour, but try not to vary it more than that.

GET UP AT THE SAME TIME EACH MORNING.
When you wake also matters. Be consistent.

DON'T SET AN ALARM.
Waking naturally is ideal if possible.

SET GENTLE ALARMS.

If you use an alarm, use a gentle-sounding alarm. A loud alarm can be fine, but the jolt is stressful. You might also want to try an alarm that wakes you up with light to mimic the sun.

DON'T NAP.

Napping is okay but should not be relied upon to complete a night's rest. Before 2 or 3 p.m., occasional napping 15 to 30 minutes is fine, if needed.

Sleep environment

GO DARK.

Make sure your bedroom is completely dark before you go to bed. Both eyes and skin detect light. Get rid of night-lights or any devices such as phone chargers or clocks that emit light. Purchase blackout curtains to help keep out streetlights or other unwanted light. A sleep mask can help if you go to sleep late, live somewhere with short summer nights, or have a partner who wakes before you.

GO QUIET.

If there is ambient noise you can't eliminate, consider investing in a white noise machine or listening to white noise on a speaker or with earbuds. You may benefit from *brown noise*, which is a deeper frequency than white.

BE COOL, BUT NOT COLD.

The ideal temperature for most is slightly cooler than their normal room temperature. The body naturally cools down at night, so a cooler temperature helps it do that. Feeling *cold* can stimulate wakefulness, but comfortably cool often helps. Hot and stuffy can keep you tossing and turning.

INVEST IN COTTON OR OTHER BREATHABLE BED LINENS.

Many synthetic fabrics trap heat and can overheat your body, leading to poor sleep, sweating, and dehydration. Make sure your mattress, pillow, blankets, and sheets are cool and comfortable throughout the night.

INVEST IN COTTON OR OTHER BREATHABLE SLEEP CLOTHES.

Sleep in pajamas that you enjoy and feel comfortable in, or no pajamas at all. Like your bedding, synthetic and other fabrics that can overheat or otherwise bother you can disrupt sleep.

INVEST IN MATTRESSES MADE OF NATURAL, BREATHABLE MATERIALS.

Mattresses can trap heat, too. Avoid foam, memory foam, or latex. These mattresses are often cheaper, but you might be paying for that with reduced sleep quality. Invest in mattresses made of natural, breathable materials. Some mattress companies now offer money-back guarantees for 30, 60, or 90 days. If you're still hot, try something new.

MINIMIZE PET DISRUPTION.

Does your pet sleep with you? Consider getting them a bed of their own and have them sleep outside your bedroom area.

MINIMIZE PARTNER DISRUPTION.

It's important to manage your sleeping relationship with any partners you share a bed with. Do they snore? Do they toss and turn all night? Talk with each other about how you can optimize your sleep. You might want to experiment with different sleeping arrangements or bed dividers. It could be worth experimenting with sleeping separately, either in the same room or different rooms, for a few days just to see the effect this has on your sleep quality and blood sugar.

Mind management

PREP TOMORROW EARLY TODAY.

Give yourself the gift of creating a feasible to-do list for tomorrow. Do it as early as you can, such as when the workday draws to a close. When you go to bed, remind yourself that you've set the tasks for tomorrow and that you already know you'll be able to accomplish them.

MEDITATE, PRAY, STRETCH, BREATHE.

Wind down well. Be intentional about it. Your body rests most easily when your mind is in a genuine state of peace. Do any favorite calming activities right before bed.

STAY RESTFUL ALL NIGHT.

If you awaken in the middle of the night, it's okay. Stay in bed. Don't get up and start doing chores. Let yourself rest. Return to your meditative practice if that helps. Lie peacefully and breathe deep. Let this be a moment of real rest. If you regularly wake in the middle of the night and feel very awake, you may be a biphasic sleeper—that is, someone who sleeps in two separate phases. In this case, you can do something productive, though not stimulating.

IF YOU CAN'T SLEEP, STAY GENTLE.

If after 20 or 30 minutes you can't sleep, try a gentle activity like knitting, listening to soothing music, or reading a book.

Body management

FINISH HYDRATING EARLY.

Finish drinking all beverages at least 2 hours before bedtime so you don't have to get up during the night to urinate.

REDUCE OR GIVE UP CAFFEINE.

Monitor how much caffeine you consume, including in all beverages, supplements, and over-the-counter drugs. Stop drinking caffeine by afternoon or consider reducing your intake or eliminating it entirely. If you aren't sure if caffeine affects your sleep, change your routine to find out. Caffeine can also elevate blood sugar, so watch your numbers when you drink it. Sources include coffee, espresso, energy drinks, black tea, green tea, white tea, chocolate, and cacao.

AVOID PROCESSED FOODS.

Processed foods, including meals provided by restaurants, usually contain high amounts of sodium, which can increase blood pressure and can contain additives such as MSG (not always required to be included on ingredient lists) that can have a stimulatory effect on the brain.

NOURISH YOURSELF WITH SUFFICIENT PROTEIN, FAT, AND CARBOHYDRATES.

Make sure you're getting a palm-size portion or cup of protein, at least a dollop of healthy fat, and your ideal portion of complex carbohydrate/resistant starch with every meal. Your body uses all three macronutrients to create the molecules and hormones it needs to fall and stay asleep.

TIME YOUR MEALS.

Eat most of your food at breakfast and/or lunch. Finish eating all food 3–5 hours before bedtime. Avoid going to bed right after eating a heavy meal.

REDUCE OR ELIMINATE ALCOHOL.
Drinking alcohol can make you feel sleepier at first, but this is sedation, not sleep. If consuming it, it's best at least 5 hours before bed.

TRY MAGNESIUM SUPPLEMENTATION.
Even people who eat healthy diets are often deficient in magnesium. Magnesium-rich foods include spinach, black beans, salmon, almonds, pumpkin seeds, pistachios, soy/edamame, peanuts, and cacao. Magnesium plays an important role in relaxing the muscles and nerves and preparing the brain for sleep. Supplementing is not a replacement for any other strategy. More information on how to supplement with magnesium and other nutrients is available in the Resources section on my website.

Exercise and stress management

NO STRESS BEFORE BED.
You can't control unpredictable events, but you can set boundaries within yourself. If there are things you know stress you out, don't do them before bed. Set a curfew on stress events: at least 90 minutes before bed. If something comes up that can be put off until the next day, put it off.

EXERCISE NEARLY DAILY, EARLY IN THE DAY.
Exercise five to seven days a week. Even a little exercise, 20 minutes each day, helps improve sleep quality and quantity. Be sure to allow at least 5 hours between your exercise and your bedtime to help your body stick to its natural rhythm.

Technology management

DON'T EMAIL BEFORE BED.

Don't check emails right before bedtime. Set a boundary for yourself and pick a time after which you don't look at email.

CURFEW YOUR SOCIAL MEDIA TIME.

Don't check social media or other messages or news feeds that might stimulate you right before bedtime. Allow at least 90 minutes between your last look at social media and bedtime.

LIMIT OR ELIMINATE NOTIFICATIONS AND OTHER GADGETS.

Don't let your sleep be interrupted by notifications or gadgets. Turn off notifications, or better yet, turn on "do not disturb" or "airplane mode." If you need to be able to receive urgent phone calls, your phone may have certain settings where designated people can reach you even if "do not disturb" is on.

SET AVAILABILITY BOUNDARIES.

Our world is hyperconnected. We are expected to be available 24 hours a day, 7 days a week. This is unnatural. Consider what boundaries you may wish to set about your own availability—via phone, text, or any messaging apps. Some families leave their phones at the door when they get home at night. Give yourself the peace and gift of presence with your family members. If setting boundaries against availability feels scary and unfamiliar to you, this might mean it's an important area to pay attention to.

SHIFT WORK: IT'S DEADLY.

The sad truth is that shift work is necessary. We do need people working the night shift. If you work nights, you're essential, and yet this rhythm is a disaster for health.

Shift work batters the body's rhythms. It disrupts important hormone and neurotransmitter production and signaling, leaving your body in the lurch and unable to carry out crucial functions. It prevents important repair processes in the brain and other organs. People who work nights are more likely to get sick, have immune dysfunction, autoimmune disease, insulin resistance, obesity, cancer, heart disease, strokes, and blood sugar dysregulation. They are also more likely to suffer from depressed or anxious moods.

Shift work reduces the ability to reset blood sugar, leading to ever-higher blood sugar numbers upon waking. In one study of male volunteers, muscular insulin sensitivity decreased after just 3.5 days of shift work.

Long-term shift work is a problematic factor in a healthy immune system, in maintaining a healthy weight, and in controlling blood sugar. Without sleep, the body stores fat more readily than it burns it.

If you work nights, zoom out and make a plan. Consider making this period of your life short-term. If you currently do shift work and have blood sugar management issues, you may not be able to leave your job right now, but I highly recommend planning to do so. Shift work is a significant obstacle to blood sugar health and can be deadly.

If you can't avoid shift work, do the best sleep hygiene you can. Eat nourishing food. Make this a top priority.

Eat a big meal when you wake up before heading to work. Your body naturally expects most of its calories early in the "day," so this can help your body approximate its natural rhythm. If you can, exercise or go for a walk around this time, too. If the sun is up, great. Go outside and enjoy it. Create as much of that "it's time to be awake!" energy as you can.

And be consistent. Try to avoid rotating shift work, which is where you change your working hours by eight hours every few weeks. This is the worst rhythm because of the inconsistency. If you can't make a change, try to have a steady shift from around 11 p.m. to 7 a.m., so you are always up in the middle of the night.

If you happen to be a rare person who prefers night work, okay. But you have to make sure at some point you see the sun. Do everything you can to get the longest and deepest sleep possible. Watch your blood sugar and for other warning signs that this is hurting your health. Be willing to make changes if your doctor advises.

SLEEP APNEA: IT CAN BE DEADLY

Sleep apnea causes you to stop breathing while you sleep, sometimes hundreds of times throughout the night, and it affects more than half of people with type 2 diabetes. This is an emergency—you're not getting oxygen! If you don't get oxygen, you die. The body enters a state of emergency. When you don't breathe at night, your body panics. It shoots adrenaline and cortisol into your blood—leading to disrupted sleep and a blood-sugar roller coaster. You might as well be running from a bear all night long.

Some of the signs include waking up with a dry mouth, a morning headache, feeling tired even after a full night's rest, snoring loudly, or episodically ceasing to breathe while you sleep.

There are two main types of sleep apnea: central and obstructive.

Central occurs when the brain fails to properly instruct the muscles that control breathing.

Obstructive is more common and caused by airway obstruction or poor airway fitness. The tongue, throat, and upper airway lack structural integrity or neuromuscular signaling when asleep, blocking the flow of air.

There are many causes of obstructive sleep apnea. One common cause is a buildup of fat around the airway, dysregulating the musculature. Carrying extra weight significantly increases the risk of sleep apnea. This can cause a vicious cycle. If excess weight causes you to develop sleep apnea, this sleep apnea increases your risk of or worsens prediabetes or type 2 diabetes. This can continue to increase weight gain.

But you can also be very lean and metabolically fit and still have sleep apnea. A thicker neck might obstruct the airway; alcohol, sedative, or other tranquilizer use can reduce muscular tone; smoking can increase inflammation and fluid retention in the upper airway; aging can contribute to a loss of muscular fitness; stress may lead to these muscles being overly tense; if you were not breastfed, you may not have developed the appropriate musculature at a critical time in infancy and early childhood.

It is quite easy to become prediabetic or diabetic due to sleep apnea. So much of the cultural discourse on type 2 diabetes today is all about how *you're lazy, you lack willpower, it's all your fault,* but sleep apnea is proof you can eat great, exercise, be lean as heck—and still develop blood sugar and insulin dysregulation because of disrupted sleep.

More than half of people with type 2 have sleep apnea. If a lover, partner, or friend says you snore or periodically cease breathing, listen to them. See a sleep doctor. Consider proper diagnostics, like a sleep study for a full assessment; this might save your life and prevent strokes and heart attacks.

Even if no one gives you such insights, consider proper diagnostic analysis anyway—especially if you don't feel well rested when you wake.

Many with sleep apnea use a *continuous positive airway pressure* (CPAP) machine, which uses air pressure to keep your airway open. CPAPs can be uncomfortable, but many of the common discomforts are avoidable if you experiment and seek out a mask size and shape that suits you. The first step to healing is getting information. The second step is acting on it. Do what you must to give yourself the long and deep sleep you need. It could save your life.

In this chapter you learned:

- Sleep matters. Lacking long and deep sleep is one of the major causes of type 2 and prediabetes.

- You can support long and deep sleep by implementing the six categories of sleep tips on pages 87–93.

- Shift work is deadly. If you must work nights, it's best only for a short time.

- Up to 50 percent of people with type 2 have sleep apnea, a dangerous sleep disorder that can cause or worsen type 2. Get tested for this, especially if you've been told you snore or periodically stop breathing while you sleep.

Quick wins/first steps:

- Go outside and get early morning light.

- Install orange light filters on your devices.

- Install blackout drapes on your windows.

- Use an eye mask, ear plugs, or a white or brown noise machine.

- Use sleep clothes, bed linens, and mattresses that enable you to stay comfortable all night.

- Set a technology curfew: no screens 90 minutes before bed. Commit to one or two weeks and see how you feel.

- Protect your peace. Set boundaries around stressful activities, social media, or communication availability before sleep.

- Reduce or eliminate caffeine.

CHAPTER 4

Exercise & Strength Training

Exercise, Especially Strength Training, Is Key.
Here's Why, and a Simple and Enjoyable Weekly Schedule

CHAPTER MAP

This chapter explains why exercise and especially
strength training fix blood sugar and heal type 2 and
prediabetes; and the chapter provides guidance for
finding the right methods for you.

KEY SECTIONS

- Active working muscles are blood sugar sponges
- The basic plan
- Strength training vs. cardio
- Personalizing workouts and making them enjoyable

Maria told me about a moment of triumph in our consultation. The Friday before, she had straightened up and wiped sweat from her brow. She had looked around and counted: 20 out of 20 boxes! Perfect: mission accomplished. Every Friday, there were about 20 boxes to unload from a food delivery truck and stack in the large pantry at the back of her Italian restaurant. But this Friday had been different: Maria had moved all 20 boxes by herself.

When she recounted this to me, she was bubbling with excitement. What a huge contrast to the frustration and despair she was feeling when I first met her.

Maria was a shorter woman, and when we first started working together, she had carried significant excess body fat. She'd tried running, but it hurt her knees. She'd tried going to the gym but felt judged. Doctors and friends all said the same: Just do more exercise, push through the exhaustion, toughen up at the gym. *She'd tried, but it was just so difficult. She blamed herself for "giving up."*

In our first meeting, I asked Maria to tell me about her experiences with exercise. "Tell me about your needs. What feels good and what doesn't? What's your schedule like?"

She told me she needed to be at the restaurant from morning to night. But she didn't want to exercise in the morning because it would cut into her precious sleep. I agreed sleep was a key priority. We brainstormed about what was feasible. We realized that she could incorporate some movement at work. She didn't have to sit behind the desk all day. She could help the staff with physical labor like stacking chairs at the end of the night and unloading deliveries. She didn't push herself to do too much at the beginning. But after a while, she started feeling stronger and more capable.

She started feeling more energetic. I could hear the smile in her voice. She also told me something wonderful: Several people on the restaurant crew had remarked to her that she had regained a long-lost spring in her step. What a beautiful thing.

In the next consultation, she told me she ordered a spin bike to put in the back office.

Amazing. Fantastic. This is what we're here to do: Find what works for you, positive change after positive change.

Sustainable fitness is all about finding the right strategy that fits your lifestyle.

ACTIVE WORKING MUSCLES ARE BLOOD SUGAR SPONGES

Exercise is marvelous for blood sugar control because active working muscles are blood sugar sponges.

When you exercise, your body burns blood sugar as fuel. As you start warming up, it starts releasing blood sugar from storage sites into your blood so it can burn it. When you're done exercising, it returns any excess sugar in the blood to the storage sites. Because you've burned through part of your body's overall sugar content, you end up with less blood sugar than when you started.

This brings two big wins.

The most immediate win is you have less blood sugar. You have a lower blood-sugar level than when you started.

The second is that this helps your cells become more insulin sensitive. Burning through blood sugar tells your cells that sugar is a little more scarce. There's a relative lack. Storage sites become more inclined to let it in.

The extent of sensitivity depends on many factors, including the intensity of exercise. Sensitivity can last a few hours after exercise. A single bout of moderate-intensity exercise can increase the movement of blood sugar into storage by 40 percent.

Active working muscles are blood sugar sponges.

THE BLOOD SUGAR HACK: GET OFF THE BLOOD-SUGAR ROLLER COASTER

One implication of this is a great gift: You can use exercise to bring down blood sugar after an unexpected spike.

If your blood sugar spikes, get up and move.

Try these:

- Do some push-ups, squats, or wall sits.

- Go for a walk or a light jog around the block.

- Go up and down your home or office stairs a few times. Maybe you can have your meetings while walking, or invite a colleague to join you if in person.

The path to healing type 2 and prediabetes lies in resetting blood sugar lower and lower. If you get in the habit of using exercise as a buffer for bad choices, you don't get as much benefit from it. The purpose of exercise is not to make up for bad blood-sugar habits. Don't sacrifice the incredible healing benefit of exercise for the sake of treats. Nothing tastes as good as healthy feels.

LONG-TERM BENEFIT

In the long-term, exercise helps boost insulin sensitivity and improves fasting blood sugar, fasting insulin, A1C, and your cholesterol profile. When you do strength training and build muscle, you multiply these benefits even further. The more muscle you have, the bigger your reservoir for sugar storage.

Exercise has also been shown to reduce inflammation and oxidative stress and improve mitochondria health, the three main types of damage to metabolic machinery. It improves anxiety and depression.

It strengthens bone density and reduces risks of heart disease, stroke, cancer, and complications and hospitalizations from illness.

EVEN WITHOUT WEIGHT LOSS

Our culture assumes a terrible myth: Weight loss is the key to health. Many think the only reason to exercise is weight loss. It's true that if you carry significant excess weight, and especially in your abdomen area around your organs, weight loss can help improve health and blood sugar. But it's a myth that the only point of exercise is to lose weight.

Recent advances in the scientific study of exercise have shown that exercise confers significant health benefits even if you don't lose weight.

A recent review concluded: Independent of weight loss, increasing physical activity was associated with about a 15–50 percent reduction in mortality. When compared to intentional weight loss, the benefits of exercise for health were more consistent and significant.

THE BASIC PLAN

- Strength train to build muscle 3 times a week.

- Exercise for at least 20–40 minutes most days (5–7 times a week).

- Keep moving throughout every day.

- Be consistent.

- Keep challenging yourself.

Strength training is uniquely beneficial for health, so if you can do it without pain or injury, then that is a priority. A starting point of 2 times a week is great; 3 times is ideal.

More isn't always better. Muscles grow through stress: Lifting heavy weights tears the muscles. Then they grow back stronger. They need time, about 24–48 hours, to repair. So get into a rhythm where you stress and rebuild, stress and rebuild.

Another priority is daily or almost-daily exercise. Do any kind of movement you enjoy for at least 20–40 minutes, 5–7 days a week. Some activities can go on for hours, like sports, hiking, or dancing. But you don't necessarily need to do more than 20–40 minutes to get good blood-sugar results.

Keep moving throughout every day. Ideally, at least 10 minutes of every hour.

Consistency is key. Find what works for you. Assess your personal level of health and capability. Meet yourself where you're at. It can take time to figure out what works best. Have grace for yourself and keep going.

If you're starting from zero, begin with whatever is feasible for you. For some, that's walking after meals, or simply some gentle stretching. Remember this is about progress, not perfection. Comparison is the thief of joy. Avoid comparing your exercise level to someone else's; celebrate the fact that you are exercising!

STRENGTH TRAINING VS. CARDIO

In general, there are two different kinds of exercise: strength training and cardio.

Strength training is when you intentionally increase your muscle strength by challenging your muscles to work against a weight or force. The most popular way to do strength training is to lift weights. You can also use weight machines, dumbbells, kettlebells, resistance bands, or your own body weight.

Cardio refers to moderate intensity over longer time periods. Things like running, biking, hiking, rowing, aerobics, kickboxing, swimming, or dancing. These all fall in the bucket of "other physical activity" that you do for at least 20 minutes, 5–7 times a week.

If you enjoy treadmills or ellipticals, vary the pace of your activity. People have called treadmills the walk of death—not because they're deadly but because they don't help all that much. You need to vary the pace for real benefit. You want your heart rate to go up and get pumping; break a sweat! Then let it come back down and get it up again.

The line between cardio and strength training is fuzzy. Cardio builds muscle, and strength training improves cardio fitness.

It's excellent to get a mix of cardio and strength training. Both are important. But when push comes to shove, strength training is a major priority. Active working muscles are blood sugar sponges, and strength training grows them. Plus, strength training helps you maintain brain health, bone health, and your proprioceptive sense, which is in charge of balance and helps prevent falls as you age.

For most of my patients, so long as there is no pain or risk of injury, and they have the capacity for it, strength training is *required*. It's common to consider weight-lifting a hobby. But the truth is that if you really want to optimize your health for the long-term, it's crucial. For the best chance of energy, health, vitality, staying upright and moving, maintaining independence, and having a strong mind and body in adulthood and your latest years? *Strength train.*

STRENGTH TRAINING IS SELF-CARE

Strength training helps you maintain your independence for as long as possible. You equip yourself for a life where you're moving and active until the end. The earlier you start, the better off you'll be. But there's no such thing as too late!

Most people are pressed for time. Life is a constant juggling act. Most people exercise only if they can fit it around everything else. *Mindset shift:* Try fitting other events around *it*. Put exercise, and especially strength training, as a priority in your schedule. Make it a habit, commit to it!

LIFT HEAVY

Muscles grow through exertion. If you don't challenge them, they don't grow.

Continue to challenge yourself by increasing the weight you lift. What's heavy for you is different from what's heavy for someone else. Judge what's heavy for you based on what feels very difficult to pick up, *while maintaining good form*, about 10 times. Let your muscles feel strain and your heart rate and breathing go up. That's natural, that's a sign you're doing it right. For different muscle groups, the amount of weight will be different.

Your biggest muscles, and likely your strongest, are in the lower body, especially your thighs. Lifting isn't just about bicep curls and the stereotypical upper body muscles you show off at the beach! You get the most benefit from a well-rounded strength training program. Take advantage of the amazing blood sugar reservoir of your lower body.

IF YOU'RE NEW TO STRENGTH TRAINING

If strength training is new, for the first two or three weeks, focus on form. Hire a personal trainer, someone to guide you, if you can. You want to perform all the movements correctly. Build a solid foundation. That way you can avoid injuries.

As you start feeling good—not so stiff and achy when you move—that's a sign you can start adding more weight. It usually happens around the third week if you're older, the second week if you're younger. You start feeling like it's not kicking your butt. You're kicking its butt! That's your signal: Progressively add more weight. Move from the very light 2- or 5-pound weights up to 8- or 10-pound weights—and keep going!

EXPLORING OPTIONS TO FIND WHAT WORKS FOR YOU

Some questions to ask yourself:

Do you enjoy your current workout routine? What haven't you tried yet that sounds fun? Do you prefer activities outdoors or indoors? Do you like seasonal activities? Do you prefer to exercise alone or in a class? What activities feel like play to you? Do you experience any feelings of empowerment or freedom?

Could you move more in the office? Take the stairs or get a standing desk? What about your commute? Could you walk or ride a bike to work?

Everybody's genes and physiology regarding exercise are different. Some get great benefits from incorporating gentle exercises like yoga or swimming. For these people, just adding walking every day on top of healthy eating patterns is what they need to get healthier in every possible way. Other people may need to lift weights or do more intense exercise. We're not the same as each other. We're also not the same at different points in our lives. Gardening or walking could be excellent for you if you're just starting out or are ninety years old. It might not make a significant difference if you're already quite active.

In the end, the best exercise for you is the one you're actually going to do.

PRO TIP: EXPERIMENT AND STAY CURIOUS, LIKE MICHAEL

Michael had never liked to exercise. He had always been heavy and unathletic, ever since he was a little kid. He had been bullied for it. As an adult he tried to change his fitness level. One year, "become a runner" was his New Year's resolution. Another year he enrolled in kickboxing. He tried joining a local gym.

None of it stuck. When he went running, he thought about all the people who would see him struggling. Plus, it hurt his knees and ankles, and when he stopped, he felt absolutely drained of energy. It always took so much willpower.

I encouraged Michael to think about what kinds of environments would make exercise less emotionally stressful for him. He thought he might enjoy the solitude and comfort of working out at home.

Michael found a personal trainer who would come to his home. He kept looking for other forms of exercise he'd enjoy. Eventually he fell in love with martial arts. That, plus his new strength training routine, gave him confidence and helped him gain energy. Alongside the improvements in sleep and stress management he was making with the Yates Protocol, he was feeling the best he'd ever felt.

PRO TIP: HARNESS WHAT FEEDS YOUR ENERGY, LIKE ERICA

Erica had never really enjoyed exercise.

When we first began working together, she didn't work out at all.

By the time of our last meeting, she was an accomplished rock climber.

How did she get from A to B? Unlike Michael, who thrived on more solitary activities, Erica was a social butterfly who felt more energized the more time she spent with people.

Erica ended up finding many welcoming fitness communities and tried a variety of group classes: spin biking, yoga, and kickboxing.

But the one that was the best fit for her was rock climbing. Many people intermingled and encouraged one another. Climbing became one of her great passions, and now she brings all her exercise-shy friends to the climbing gym to try it out.

TRY HIGH-INTENSITY INTERVAL TRAINING (HIIT)

HIIT involves short bursts of high-intensity exercise. You vary your heart rate on purpose: increasing it up to 80 percent of your max, then back down. For example, you could alternate between 2 minutes of high-intensity spinning and 2 minutes at a gentle pace.

HIIT can work well for some because it doesn't take much time, and there's often a big payoff for blood sugar control. Because you get your heart rate up high, you need to perform it only for 20 minutes. People often do HIIT on stationary bikes, in spin class, on ellipticals, on treadmills, or while out running or rowing.

If you're entirely new to fitness or HIIT, try a class or session with a trainer who can guide you on the appropriate intervals and exercises for you. You'll likely want to start out low and slow. At the beginning, your high-intensity interval might be just 10 seconds of sprinting, paired with 1 minute of walking. Over time, increase the length of the high-intensity intervals. Meet yourself where you're at, then keep challenging yourself more and more.

HIIT is pretty demanding, so it's not for everybody. But the body makes feel-good neurotransmitters when you do it, and many rate HIIT as more enjoyable than steady-state cardio.

HIIT may also be more effective than steady-state cardio for shedding visceral abdominal fat, which is the fat that is the most dangerous for type 2 and prediabetes. Additionally, it's been shown to improve depression more than steady-state cardio.

If you feel good doing HIIT, it can be incorporated 3 or 4 times a week.

WHEN—FIND YOUR DAYS AND TIMES

The best days to exercise and strength train are days where you are actually going to do it!

In my clinical experience, many people like a rhythm of strength training on Wednesday and Saturday. Mondays are often too busy. Wednesdays are often a win because people like the boost of energy to propel them over the hill of the week. That pairs well with a weekend day like Saturday.

Just stay curious and see what works! If one rhythm doesn't feel sustainable to you, try a different one.

Time of day also matters.

One great time for many people is first thing in the morning before breakfast. This is called exercising fasted. It can help with blood sugar control, especially if you wake up with an exaggerated dawn phenomenon (page 83). It helps with fat burning, especially that visceral abdominal fat. People who exercise in a fasted state often find they have a much easier time controlling their weight, metabolism, and mood.

You may prefer exercising after breakfast or lunch if you want to bring your blood sugar levels back down after a meal, or if you like a bump of energy in the afternoons. If you have type 1 diabetes, this may be ideal, as you need to have sufficient sugar in your blood.

Test your blood sugar immediately after exercise, then an hour later. Check it the next morning as soon as you wake up. Is it better than normal? And ask yourself: Do I feel more energized? Do I feel like my mood is more even? Is my blood pressure better? It's all good information.

It's important to allow plenty of time between exercise and sleep. Make sure you get your exercise done by the mid- to late afternoon. If you must exercise in the evening, that's okay, but avoid it within 5 hours of sleep; 3 is the absolute *minimum*. Exercise causes a boost in the stress/wakefulness hormone cortisol, so late exercise can throw off your circadian rhythm and all the good body/clock synchrony you've achieved through good sleep hygiene and meal timing. Nighttime is when your body wants cortisol to be going down. Give your brain, gut, and muscles the gift of being able to work together.

FIND YOUR FEASIBLE WHERE AND WITH WHAT

Location matters. Many people think they have to go to a gym to exercise, and for some, that works; but for others, it's just not appealing. Plus, the amount of time and energy it takes to get there can be prohibitive. What if there's traffic? What if it's raining? If you always feel motivated to go, great. Do it. But some find the act of getting the clothes, the gym bag, trekking to the gym, setting up at a locker, etc., to be too much.

If you stay home, invest in the equipment you need. For an effective workout routine, you need less than you might think at first glance. Technically, if you do push-ups, squats, and wall sits, you don't need anything other than yourself. Adding weights will help. You can purchase single sets of dumbbells or a kettlebell if you're just starting out. Consult a trainer on what would be best for a beginner's home gym.

KEEP MOVING

Perhaps most important of all is to keep moving.

Most people wake up, eat, get in their cars, sit in an office all day long, eat, drive home, sit down, eat, and go to sleep. Our culture is possibly the most sedentary in history. According to the American Heart Association, sedentary jobs have increased by 83 percent since 1950.

A sedentary way of life is deadly.

Sitting for long periods has been referred to as the "sitting disease." Some say *sitting is the new smoking*. It's true. Even daily exercise doesn't make up for the deadliness of sitting for the other 23 hours. Among those who exercise regularly, sitting for long periods is associated with worse health outcomes. including type 2 diabetes, heart disease, and cancer.

Ideally, you're moving 10 minutes of every hour. It could be cleaning around the house, doing some chores, or walking around the block. Set a timer to remind you to get up and do 10 squats, a few push-ups, or dance to your favorite song.

If at work, change the "smoke break" to a "movement break." Familiarize yourself with your building's stairs and, if reasonable, always take them, no excuses! Get up and walk around the office, say hi to some colleagues, take a little trip down to the first floor and back up. I keep a kettlebell under my desk and do a few kettlebell swings between Zoom calls.

Standing up while you work or using a treadmill desk are great options. If you can't get away from your desk, consider swapping your chair for an exercise ball. Bouncing on the exercise ball can actually reduce a blood sugar spike after a meal. It's best to get up and move, but these little interventions can help in a pinch.

WALK AFTER MEALS

Many cultures around the world encourage regular walking after meals. I like the Chinese saying, *Fan ou bai bu zou huo dao jiu shi jiu*: "If you take 100 steps after each meal, you'll live to 99." There's even a word for the post-meal walking in Italian: *passeggiata*. People have known for a long time that this is important.

Today there is plenty of science to back up this activity. Walking after eating is associated with elevated mood, smoother digestion, steadier blood sugar, and increased circulation, boosting both energy and mental clarity. Even 10 minutes shows improvements.

This is an excellent way to keep yourself moving and help blunt a blood sugar rise after meals at the same time. Making this a regular habit can go a long way.

KEY POPULATIONS: IT'S ESPECIALLY
IMPORTANT AS YOU AGE

Many mistakenly think it's natural to move less as you age. You're *supposed* to become inactive. You're *supposed* to have less muscle mass. While true that aging entails a general and gentle decline of most body functions, it's not nearly as set in stone as we make it out to be.

Today, people are living longer than ever before, but the quality of life at the end has decreased. About 30 percent of American adults over seventy-five have trouble with walking, getting out of a chair, or climbing stairs. Everyday tasks are more difficult. Falls are more likely. Nursing home admission is more likely. Being in a walker or wheelchair is more likely.

The truth is humans can be vital movers throughout life, until the end of life.

The key to this is doing all five steps of the Yates Protocol, and exercise especially.

Exercise isn't *less* important as you age, but *more*. It's not *less* important to move often, but *more*. Not *less* important to lift weights, but *more*.

You must preserve your muscle mass as you age. It helps with balance, coordination, and proprioception (the sense that manages communication between your inner ear and brain and helps you not fall). Falling is often the beginning of a cycle of poorer health and premature death. Strength train. No matter your age, you can incorporate some form of activity now. Give yourself the gifts of capability and vitality later in life. Preserve your independence and personal autonomy.

PRO TIP: PRIORITIZE SAFETY AND WORK WITH TRUSTED HELP, LIKE EDNA

My patient Edna began weight-lifting as a senior citizen. She had never lifted weights before. She wanted to do it right to lay the foundation of her future health.

"I'm ready to match my physical strength to my inner strength, Dr. Yates!" she said.

Edna found a personal trainer who could guide her on her form. Some gyms offer discounts or free consultations when you get started. She found help that fit her budget. Edna worked with a trainer for a month while she figured out how to lift safely. She continued on her own, but any time she had a question about what was safe, she asked it. This enabled her to keep lifting heavier and heavier weights, and to support her bone health and balance and avoid falls as she grew older. It also significantly improved her blood sugar control.

Last time I saw Edna, she told me she felt younger and more energetic than she had in years. She felt empowered in a way she had never understood before. She was glad she had taken the leap to get started and continued to challenge herself, all while prioritizing her safety and health.

KEY POPULATIONS: WOMEN—LIFT WEIGHTS!

Our culture stigmatizes women who lift weights. This is sad. If you think women shouldn't weight lift or they look weird with muscles, I invite you to get curious about why that's so. There may be cultural biases standing in the way of your doing something fabulous for yourself.

One study of more than 35,000 women from forty-seven to ninety-two years old showed that those who did strength training as a part of their exercise regimens had a 30 percent lower rate of type 2 diabetes than those who did not strength train.

Osteoporosis affects 10 million Americans, and 80 percent of them are women. Half of all women over fifty will eventually develop osteoporosis. This significantly increases the risk of breaking bones. You can help defend against this by incorporating strength training into your weekly routine. If you already have osteoporosis or are on the way there with the precursor condition of osteopenia, you can fight back now by lifting weights.

Older women especially grew up in a world where *women just didn't strength train.* If you're an older woman, pumping iron may be unfamiliar to you. But it is incredibly beneficial, fun, feels great, keeps you strong and steady, and is not at all as difficult as it may seem.

If you're a woman fifty or older, you should strength train 3 times a week, and don't be afraid to lift heavy. In your first 2–3 weeks, focus on getting the form down. Then pick up some light dumbbells. Then increase the weight over time. Put some pressure on. If you think about women's roles all over the world, we're not going to break! We're not fragile like that, not even as we age, not even if we have more porous bones. Challenge yourself with your fitness. Cultivate physical fitness to match your already fierce inner fitness.

KEY POPULATIONS: IF YOU'RE IN PAIN, INJURED, DEPRESSED, EXHAUSTED, OR JUST NOT READY, THEN EXERCISE IS OPTIONAL

Exercise is marvelous. It's required if you can do it. But if you can't, it's not *abandon all hope ye who enter here.* The way society frames it: *If you're not exercising, you're a worthless piece of scum and won't get better.* People internalize this. Some conclude: *Oh God, if I can't exercise, I'm toast.*

This is not true. I've seen people hold the line on blood sugar disasters and even turn their health around without exercising at first.

The people who succeed doing this eat reasonably well, pay attention to meal timing, and are working on their sleep or stress. If you've got at least three of the other four steps of the Yates Protocol in good order, you're improving. You can return to exercise later, as soon as you feel ready and are cleared by your doctor.

Meet Pam.

When I began working with Pam, she'd had type 2 for over twenty-five years. She was not in a good situation: sedentary, craving crackers and what she now calls "crapola," very low energy, exhausted and fatigued all the time, depressed.

We started with supplementation for mitochondrial support. This can help provide a boost of energy. Three consultations and six weeks later, she was able to get off the couch because of this mitochondrial support. Then we moved to her nutrition. She steadily incorporated more leafy greens and less crapola. She started craving more natural food. It happened naturally as she gained energy and began to heal her underlying systems. Three-bean salad became her favorite! She began reducing snacks.

After a couple of months, she began intentional physical fitness at home. This was a big win.

Then, she returned to her gym. She hired a personal trainer. Today, she exercises 4–5 days a week.

In the middle of all this, some unexpected crises befell Pam's life all at once. Two dear family members passed away. Two friends needed help in different parts of the country. She drove quite a distance to help these friends. Throughout that whole ordeal, she kept taking care of herself. This is such a big win for someone who's had the disease for twenty-five-plus years, and who's vulnerable to depression.

Many at those points throw up their hands, *I'm done, I'm cooked.*

But Pam had slowly built habits that supported her health. Bit by bit. Step by step. And she was able to keep going and going.

Today, Pam is still going. She is at her healthiest weight in forty-four years, has halved her prescriptions for cholesterol and depression, is no longer on over-the-counter medications for her stomach, and has her energy levels back. Her most recent A1C reading was 5.6. That's full-on reversal of type 2 diabetes, and she consistently exercises and is walking 3 miles 4–5 days a week.

For some people, getting out of bed is the big win. We have to honor that. Let's celebrate that. Health is about making progress, not meeting some arbitrary standard, a picture of fitness that isn't accessible to you or right for you—at this stage in your life, or any stage.

If you're in pain, have recently been in surgery, or are taking corticosteroids or certain other medications, this will raise your blood sugar. Just pain by itself can raise blood sugar if it feels stressful enough. Exercise can help with high blood sugar, but it's more effective to prioritize healing. Don't force yourself to run before you can walk. Let your body recover from these stressors. Work with a health-care practitioner to figure out what might be best for you in such circumstances. And have grace for yourself and your body as you find your way.

I'm not telling you to ignore exercise. It's helpful. It's important. But if you're in pain, if you're injured, if you're depressed, exhausted, if you *can't* bring yourself to do it, okay. Don't sweat the fact that you're unable to do it right now. You will likely be able to do it later. Focus on what's feasible and accessible to you, what can help you heal. Do the other steps of the Yates Protocol. It's possible you will be like Pam in your own way, regaining capacities for movement and fitness as you keep taking more steps on this path.

You know yourself well. You know what you're capable of. It's important to be honest with yourself and to look for solutions. Sometimes certain kinds of pain and injury can be worked around. Say you're quite heavy, and standing hurts your knees. You have some options: You could get in the pool, or you could do upper body exercises sitting down. These both take the pressure off your knees. Find a way to take that pressure off. Try a rowing machine. Do gentle stretches. Start where you are. Keep going one day at a time.

If you're experiencing chronic pain, seek out help: Explore medications, acupuncture, supplements, physical therapy.

But sometimes it may not go away. What do you do? Be patient with yourself and support your health. This likely means finding a way to exercise in spite of the pain.

My mom had rheumatoid arthritis. I don't know how people with rheumatoid arthritis get through their days with the grinding, incessant pain. She was most days probably at a 12 or 15 out of 10 on a pain scale. But no matter how difficult her circumstances, she kept incorporating movement into her day. She was going to be in pain whether she was moving or not, so she chose to get up and live her life to the fullest. She knew if she didn't keep moving, it was going to be worse as she aged. She stayed active her whole life.

Take it day by day. There's no need to push yourself unduly. The goal is *better*, and the most potent source of better is *healing*. Heal yourself in realistic and sustainable ways.

TYING IT TOGETHER: EXERCISE WITH OTHER STEPS

Exercise has a great relationship with all the other steps of the Yates Protocol.

For nutrition, it's important to continue to eat well. Sometimes people go crazy with food after working out, piling their plates high with "post-workout carbs" like pasta or pizza. They justify it as post-workout carbs. No. It doesn't work like that. You can't out-exercise a bad diet. Your body is made from what you eat.

Many of my patients experience reduced cravings for junk foods when they begin to exercise. The more you incorporate movement into your life, the more you crave nutrition that helps you perform it. Exercise also helps improve the balance between the hormones ghrelin and leptin, setting your natural hunger and satiation signals back on track.

When it comes to both meal timing and sleep, exercise should *support*, not *hinder*, your natural rhythm. Exercise typically improves sleep, especially when done earlier in the day. Many who exercise report that their sleep noticeably improves. One element of falling and staying asleep is the production of adenosine, a molecule produced while awake that creates "sleep pressure." Exercise stimulates extra adenosine production.

Exercise helps with stress. Regular exercise supports healthy neurotransmitter production and blood sugar balance. Many use exercise to stay mentally and emotionally on track. Some of my patients tell me part of the reason they stick to their exercise regimens is that it helps them feel calmer or motivated each day.

Exercise can also be a great tool for stress management in the immediate moment. If you experience stress, anxiety, or even boredom, throw on your sneakers and do some kettlebell swings or go for a walk outside. It can help burn off the cortisol and amplify good feeling neurotransmitters in the brain.

Exercise is not a cure-all for any difficulties with mood, anxiety, or depression, but it is an area where the quality of life is absolutely improved.

EXERCISE AND BLOOD SUGAR NUMBERS

Blood sugar rises when you exercise. This is natural. Sugar is released from muscles and other storage sites in order to be burned. It can rise especially high with intense exercise, since there's more demand for energy and therefore more sugar released. But this is temporary. Do not panic. If you wear a continuous glucose monitor (CGM), be patient and watch. It should reset within about an hour.

Use your CGM (or glucometer) to monitor your blood sugar rise and fall before, during, and after your workout. If you have a glucometer, test yourself immediately before and after a workout, then an hour later. Does it reset down to a lower level than when you started? That's great news, exactly what you want to see.

You can experiment to see about getting those resetting numbers even lower. Try different types of workouts: HIIT, cardio, playing sports, lifting weights. Vary length and intensity. Track your numbers in a notebook and see what works best for you.

You also want to look at the potential impact of exercise on the rest of your day. Do your blood sugar numbers reset better after meals? If you exercise in the morning, you may see better resetting after breakfast or lunch, for example. And how are your numbers when you wake up the next day?

Just getting moving is a big win. But to amplify your healing and success, use that precious blood sugar data. *Test, don't guess.*

GET STARTED: 5 GUIDELINES TO GETTING THE MOST OUT OF EXERCISE

1. Safety first. Avoid falling and injury.
2. Choose feasible activities.
3. Choose enjoyable activities.
4. Choose activities good for your personal blood-sugar control and health.
5. Find your rhythm.

In this chapter you learned:

- The basic exercise plan is:

  - Strength train 2–3 times a week,

  - Exercise for at least 20–40 minutes most days (5–7 days a week),

  - Incorporate movement throughout the day,

  - Be consistent,

  - Keep challenging yourself.

- Active working muscles are blood sugar sponges.

- Exercise increases insulin sensitivity in the short- and long-term. Regular exercise boosts health in many ways, including improving blood sugar control and insulin sensitivity. Give yourself this gift.

- Strength training is especially beneficial because it grows muscle, strengthens bones, supports brain health, and helps prevent falls.

- Exercise and strength training become *more*, not less, important as you age.

- Sitting is deadly. Get up every hour for 10 minutes.

- Everybody's fitness needs are different. Meet yourself where you are.

- Pain and exhaustion or depression are barriers to exercise. If you can't yet exercise, focus on healing yourself until you can.

Quick wins/first steps:

- If you're a beginner, get in touch with a gym or trainer to help you perfect your basic form and write a training plan that works for your needs.

- Identify the best days and times for you to strength train. Pick at least 2 days a week. Block it off in your calendar. Commit to it for at least a month.

- Pick a new activity to try. Try it for one month. If you don't like it after that time, try something else. Experiment!

- Add a 10-minute walk after dinner for 1 week.

- Look for opportunities to integrate more movement into your daily life: taking the stairs, carrying groceries, vacuuming, walking while on the phone or in work meetings.

- When experiencing a blood sugar spike, get up and move.

CHAPTER 5

Stress

It's the Cause of Type 2 and Prediabetes No One Talks About.
Use These 3 Strategies to Fight Back and Win

CHAPTER MAP

This chapter explains the devastating effects of stress on blood sugar and provides three management strategies.

KEY SECTIONS

- Life in Cortisol Nation
- Stress: A key cause of unhealthy behaviors
- STRATEGY 1: Manage stress triggers
- STRATEGY 2: Establish healthy habits
- STRATEGY 3: Incorporate stress-reducing practices into daily life

Sandra emerged from the subway onto the street and checked her watch. She hefted her bag more firmly over her shoulder and strode across the street. She'd stayed an extra two hours at work, but that was the norm these days, and she didn't have time to worry about it. She needed to get home ASAP. Her mother had another round of tests at the hospital tonight. Will we ever get a break? *She sighed. She had to pick up some of her things, then hurry to the hospital. Maybe she'd take a few minutes to grab a bite to eat.*

She might not have the time for candlelit baths or to cook for herself, but she could at least take some time to change into more comfortable clothes.

As Sandra strode down the street, she felt her eyelids drooping. It was too late for another coffee, but maybe she could get away with a diet soda. She rarely slept more than five hours a night these days. Had she eaten today? *Oh yeah, the bagel. She'd had one and an orange juice. She was a little cautious about drinking too much juice because she was prediabetic, but her blood sugar readings had been stable for years. Her prediabetes was another one of those* totally fine *things.*

Sandra was about to push her front door open when she got an email notification on her phone. She paused with one foot on the porch. She shifted her weight to her other foot and let her purse drop to the ground. Oh! It was test results from her doctor's office. She opened the email, then paused.

Oh.

Oh.

6.6.

For years, *Sandra's A1C had stayed steady at 5.8. Now her A1C was 6.6.*

She wasn't just prediabetic anymore. She had full-blown type 2. It hit her like a ton of bricks. She sat down on the steps and just stared at her phone. She buried her head in her hands and began to cry. She was already doing three people's jobs at work, caring for her ailing mom, sleeping five hours a night . . . How could she add type 2 diabetes *to all this?*

She would later say to me: "I wish I could have paid more attention to me. *I'm sure my body was waving, saying 'Hey, over here, what about us?' I kept finding ways to keep going: more coffee, more breakroom food . . . without pausing to take care of myself or look for an underlying cause. I thought, 'Prediabetes, what's the big deal?' But when you take that little* 'pre' *off, ouch."*

LIFE IN CORTISOL NATION

Today, stress is the norm. Whether it's to perform at work, to manage a household, to take care of children or ailing family members . . . We're always under pressure. Few of us ever feel we have enough time to do it all. It seems like our to-do lists go on for miles. Check something off it, and more things just pile on. Always going, always rushing, always managing . . . *something.*

Always "on" is typical. Scrambling to hold it all together is typical.

But there is a problem: It's not *natural.* We were designed for a different rhythm of life.

Today, many of us walk slowly only on vacation. Think about that. On a normal day, you might, like hundreds of millions of others, wake with a jolt of alarm to an alarm clock. You might then hurriedly make coffee to take on the go, sit in bumper-to-bumper traffic, willing it to go faster—or squeeze yourself onto standing-room-only subway cars—to spend the day in an office rushing to meet deadlines, and then finally go home exhausted, mentally preparing yourself to do it all again the next day. On top of this, you live under threats of termination, of taxes, of bills, of various responsibilities, and of dangers in the world, on local and global scales.

Cortisol is the body's main stress hormone. It keeps us awake and powers us through challenges that come our way. It's the hormone of *Let's go! Time to take care of things!* It's the body's on button.

We live in Cortisol Nation, where everything is usually stuck in the on position.

I remember when I was a child. In the US, most businesses were closed on Sundays, and no one was on their work email. Now in Cortisol Nation, it's 24/7 of go, go, go. And really, where are we going?

We are supposed to live primarily in the off condition, and then to occasionally turn on.

But in Cortisol Nation, we're so on, it's difficult even to imagine what it's like to live primarily in the off mode. Off is a luxury—it's *vacation*. Think of all the words we use when we go on vacation: *time off, day off, turning off, shutting off, off the grid, out of office*.

We all know this is a problem. But everyone's doing it, right? Like Sandra, we keep pushing because we see no other choice. We don't prioritize ourselves, because we *can't*, or we feel that we can't. When it comes to listening to and taking care of our bodies, the norm in our culture is to just keep putting it off and pushing through.

We say things like "What doesn't kill you only makes you stronger," "Steel sharpens steel," and "You have to pressurize coal to make a diamond." It's true that some kinds of stress can be good for you and growth happens through adversity.

But the reality is that occasional adversity is different from living under the incessant demands of Cortisol Nation.

And the reality is that stress is physical, not just mental, in its impact.

The truth is that what doesn't kill you in Cortisol Nation . . . well, it can have long-term effects that will kill you later on. Stress is deadly serious.

In the first half of this chapter, I outline the serious effects that stress has on the body. In the second half, I share stress management strategies I've developed after decades of researching and refining approaches with my patients. There are three main prongs: managing triggers of stress, establishing healthy habits, and incorporating stress-reducing practices into daily life.

STRESS, SUPERHERO MODE, AND TYPE 2 AND PREDIABETES

The stress our ancestors experienced was rarer, but intense. A sudden rainstorm might create a flash flood. A pride of lions might circle camp. They lived in relative peace, and without smartphones, but also needed to be able to go from sleeping to hurling a spear at a moment's notice.

They developed—and we inherited—the ability to switch into what I call "superhero mode." When you detect a threat, your body pumps adrenaline and cortisol into the bloodstream, which trigger several physiological changes that prepare you for intense physical action: Your heart speeds up, your brain develops laser-like focus, your muscles tense. *And*, because blood sugar is the fuel that muscles burn, blood sugar is released into the bloodstream.

This system worked great for our ancestors. They needed this surge of blood sugar so they could run or fight off predators. They were responding to actual immediate threats. When they were safe, the threat would be over. They would go sit by the campfire and let their bodies calm down. They'd switch out of superhero mode.

The system doesn't work well for us in this modern era.

Most of us are in some state of superhero mode all the time. Every time you detect a potential threat, your body prepares you for a physically demanding emergency. It doesn't matter what the threat is. It could be the subject line of an email, or a call from your mother-in-law. Your body is going to react as if you've seen a lion: muscles tensing, heart pumping, cortisol causing sugar to flood into your bloodstream.

And then—you probably just sit there. You just sit there, maybe at your desk, or in a cubicle, with your heart pumping excess sugar around your body as hard and fast as it can.

Your body scrambles to bring the blood sugar levels back down. Your pancreas secretes high volumes of insulin to grab blood sugar and put it back in storage sites. This often works, but at a cost: a crash. It's unpleasant. You haven't done any physically exhausting work, but your organs have. So, you feel tired, and you're sluggish. Another possible outcome is the body doesn't succeed in getting blood sugar to come down quickly, and blood sugar and insulin just remain high.

The immediate panic may have passed, but often the perceived threat persists. So, your body stays in superhero mode and keeps making cortisol. Blood sugar keeps flooding out of storage sites into the blood. Your pancreas keeps racing to make insulin to put the blood sugar back in the storage sites. You might crash again. The continued presence of cortisol in your blood stimulates the release of blood sugar from storage sites again. And insulin rises to chase it back into them.

This is a blood-sugar roller coaster. It's unpleasant. And it plays a role in causing type 2 and prediabetes.

NEGATIVE HEALTH EFFECTS OF THE BLOOD-SUGAR ROLLER COASTER

The roller coaster plays a key role in the development of type 2 and prediabetes.

One reason is that it's exhausting to the pancreas. The beta cells that produce insulin in the pancreas are already under siege from inflammation and oxidative stress (pages 233–34). Demanding more work from them exhausts their capabilities.

Second, high blood sugar is inflammatory. As I explain more in chapter 9, excess sugar is sticky in the presence of inflammation. The way it sticks to other molecules results in the creation of destructive and inflammatory molecules called *advanced glycation end products* (AGEs). AGEs tear apart the tissues they touch. They are one of the most dangerous sources of damage to metabolic machinery, causing inflammation, blocking insulin from doing its job, and damaging the cells in the pancreas that produce insulin.

Third, cortisol signals to the body to shut down functions that it deems nonessential to immediate survival. These include key parts of the digestive, endocrine, and immune systems that are necessary to maintain metabolic and overall health.

Finally, constantly being in superhero mode has one other super-powerful, very negative influence on health that almost no one talks about, which does everybody with type 2 and prediabetes another injustice:

Stress changes the brain and hormones in ways that may increase your desire to make unhealthy choices.

STRESS: A KEY CAUSE OF UNHEALTHY BEHAVIORS

Most of us know that stress makes us more likely to make bad choices. Risky or unhealthy activities like staying up all night, going to the bar after work, skipping workouts, smoking, gambling, retail therapy, mindless snacking, bingeing on unhealthy foods . . . We're more likely to do them when we're stressed.

What we misunderstand is *why*.

It's not because we're lazy, or weak, or self-indulgent. It's not just because it's easier or more convenient. The convenience is part of it, of course. But at its root it's because of something even more powerful:

Superhero mode *provokes physiological changes in the brain and body* that make you more likely to make unhealthy choices.

Remember: Stress is a *physical* event.

Here are just a few of the physical changes that happen:

First, stress changes your brain to make you more impulsive.

Excess cortisol deteriorates the area of the brain called the prefrontal cortex, which is responsible for making and executing rational decisions. Your prefrontal cortex is owed thanks for the kinds of decisions you likely consider smart or healthy, like calling your mom instead of your ex or choosing salad over pizza. Cortisol, however, reduces pre-frontal firing and connectivity. This impairs your ability both to think rationally and to execute rational decisions, making you more likely to call your ex or choose the pizza.

Simultaneously, the part of the brain that specializes in emotional processing, the amygdala, grows stronger. The amygdala is instinctive and impulse driven. It's exactly the kind of decision-maker you need when there's a lion prowling and you must act fast. But it is not well suited to life in Cortisol Nation. Today, it makes you more likely to act on impulse. When you're always in superhero mode, this really makes a difference.

Second, chronic stress depletes many key nutrients necessary for mental health. One example is magnesium.

Magnesium plays an important role in more than three hundred reactions in the body, including helping nerves and muscles switch off after stress. When magnesium is low, they can get stuck in the "on" position, leaving your muscles tense and nerves running hot. A lack of magnesium can lead to serotonin depletion and damage neurons, pro-gressing to deteriorated mental health and predispositions to anxiety and depression. Lacking magnesium can also cause insomnia and anxiety, since magnesium is necessary for the brain to produce melatonin—the molecule that puts you to sleep—and GABA (gamma-aminobutyric acid)—the primary inhibitory (calming) molecule re-sponsible for inhibiting brain excitability. Without magnesium, we are much more likely to be worn down by sleepless nights and sad and anxious thoughts. (For more on magnesium supplementation, see the Resources section on the website.)

Finally, stress messes with the hormones that regulate appetite, what I call the twin gremlins ghrelin and leptin. Ghrelin makes you feel hungry. Leptin makes you feel full. Stress knocks them out of balance, so appetite-regulating mechanisms go haywire. You can de-velop a strong, even overpowering, desire to overeat. You may even consciously know in the moment that you are overeating and continue to do it anyway. You may not feel like you're in control. You might fight it throughout the day and into the evening—and then at night just binge.

This cycle weakens your ability to make peace with food.

Worse, the food you crave is the unhealthiest of the lot. This is unfortunate—but it makes evolutionary sense. Foods high in fat and sugar provide energy, which the body once needed for killing lions and other predators.

The difficulty of resisting these foods is compounded by the world we live in. When our ancestors lived off the land, and even when our grandparents just made food at home, the amount of reward they could get from food was limited. Foods could be *delicious*, but they stayed delicious *on a human level*. Today, with billions in corporate profits at stake and food scientists distorting food-like ingredients to stimulate desire for ultra-processed junk foods, foods have gained an almost superhuman power over us.

A Snickers bar, for example, is extremely strategically engineered. As you chew it, the sugar dissolves, the fat melts, and the caramel traps the peanuts in a specifically formulated order, so the combo of flavors hits your tongue just right. It creates a very powerful feeling of reward in your brain—more powerful than the brain was designed to handle. When stressed, and with the hormones of hunger and satiety ghrelin and leptin misfiring, the allure of this reward is overwhelmingly strong.

The *convenience* of modern food compounds the issue. Stress usu-ally makes us choose more convenient foods. The idea, of course, is that it'll save time or energy. But convenience comes at a steep cost: It decreases the amount of satisfaction you can get from food.

Dopamine is a neurotransmitter involved in the feeling of reward. People often talk about the "hit of dopamine" you get when you eat something tasty. That's true—you do get a little hit of dopamine. But dopamine is better understood as a molecule of reward from *seeking*. It's not the physical pleasure of eating so much as the seeking and ob-taining a pleasurable thing to eat. The implication is profound: The more effort you put into getting something—including a meal—the more intrinsically rewarding it is. That is, when you go to the drive-through, you may likely end up less satisfied than if you'd cooked at home, even if the drive-through food was really, really tasty.

We assume that convenience helps us. We lean on it in times of stress. But readily available foods—whether grabbed through a window or dropped on your doorstep—actually decrease your ability to be satisfied by food. Convenience is yet another wolf in sheep's clothing of the modern food industry.

UNHEALTHY CHOICES RECAP: *IT'S NOT YOUR FAULT!*

In summary, constant stress of superhero mode:

- degrades rational thinking and acting in the brain;

- shifts decision-making power to the amygdala, which relies on emotion and instinct;

- depletes magnesium, which is crucial for relaxation and mental health;

- imbalances ghrelin and leptin, which are necessary for healthy appetite;

- makes you the prey of those who profit off hijacking your appetite.

Going off the rails? Craving chips? Wanna skip your workout? It's not your fault.

Write it on your hand. Scrawl it on your mirror with lipstick. Put it on a sticky note on your desk. *It's not your fault.*

Stress is a physical event with physical effects. It puts you on a blood-sugar roller coaster and makes you more likely to fall into unhealthy choices and habits.

The good news is you can do something about it.

Is stress the cause of type 2 and prediabetes?

According to the National Institute of Diabetes and Digestive and Kidney Diseases, the three causes of type 2 and prediabetes are "overweight, obesity, and physical inactivity." It adds, "The location of body fat also makes a difference" because "extra belly fat is linked to insulin resistance, type 2 diabetes, and heart and blood vessel disease." Other recognized experts recommend a severely restricted diet—just 700 or 800 calories a day—to help people with type 2 and prediabetes lose significant amounts of weight quickly. They say this is because type 2 diabetes is caused by too much fat inside the liver and the pancreas, which prevents the organs from functioning as they should.

These approaches have some truth to them. When people who carry excess visceral fat around their organs lose some of it, they typically (at least in the short term) improve their fasting blood sugar, fasting insulin, and A1C levels. But that isn't the whole picture. Globally, the majority of people with type 2 diabetes are slender when diagnosed. One study of some 10,000 people with type 2 diabetes in India revealed that 63 percent of people had "ideal body weight" at diagnosis. This significantly questions any assumption that body fatness is the sole or primary cause of type 2 and prediabetes.

The real underlying cause is damage to metabolic machinery. This machinery includes many interlocking systems and organs: the gut and its microbiome, the immune system, the liver, fat and muscle cells, the pancreas, the cardiovascular system, and the nervous system.

Here is a selection of some of the ways stress damages metabolic machinery and contributes to the development of type 2 and prediabetes:

1. Cortisol stimulates sugar to be released into the bloodstream. High blood sugar contributes to systemic inflammation via the production of AGEs (advanced glycation end products) and other harmful by-products.

2. The blood-sugar roller coaster exhausts the pancreas.

3. Cortisol inhibits the production of mucus in the gut, which is there to coat the bowel wall and help keep digestion regular. Without regular bowel movements, toxins can more easily be reabsorbed into the bloodstream. This is highly inflammatory.

4. Decreased intestinal mucus changes the chemical environment, which makes it more difficult for good bacteria to thrive and easier for bad bacteria to take over. Good bacteria neutralize toxins and help prevent them from passing through the intestinal walls. When good bacteria die off and bad bacteria multiply, the weakened defenses and increased toxic load strain the immune system and cause systemic inflammation.

5. Superhero mode causes the immune system to initiate processes related to acute inflammation, such as wound healing. It produces pro-inflammatory cytokines meant to create inflammation at the site of wounds (responsible for such things as swelling and redness around a cut). This helps deliver resources to the wounds for healing and is great for acute injuries. But when cytokines are out of balance and remain too high for too long, they contribute to chronic, systemic inflammation, driving insulin resistance and type 2 and prediabetes.

6. Stress depletes nutrients' helpful blood sugar management. I already mentioned magnesium's role in stress and sleep, but another danger of low magnesium is that it's been shown to impede enzymes related to glucose metabolism and insulin receptor function.

7. Stress impairs sleep. Sleep is a critical time for resetting

blood sugar levels and replenishing the metabolic machinery.

8. Stress interferes with appetite hormone signaling. When ghrelin and leptin are out of balance, it can become nearly impossible for you to experience proper fullness signals, leading to runaway cravings and eating.

9. Stress changes brain chemistry and function, reducing the likelihood of healthy choices.

10. Stress increases the likelihood of developing visceral fat around the abdominal organs. Visceral fat secretes inflammatory molecules, contributing to type 2 and other inflammatory conditions.

So:

Is stress *the* cause of type 2 and prediabetes?

No. Stress is not *the* primary cause for *every* person. Every person's experience is unique. But it *can* be the primary cause for some people.

And it matters for everybody. Failing to take stress seriously as a cause of type 2 does all people with type 2 or prediabetes an injustice.

STRESS IS A BULLY—BUT YOU'RE FAR FROM POWERLESS

In over thirty years of working with patients, I've seen people regain blood sugar control and get their health back, even in the highest-stress situations you can imagine.

For example, Sandra started taking stress management and other aspects of the Yates Protocol seriously. She uses an app to calculate what her A1C is projected to be, based on her fasting morning blood-sugar numbers. As of this writing, she has shifted her type 2 down into prediabetic ranges (from an A1C of 6.6 to an A1C of 6.1); this is called remission. I anticipate her numbers will keep going down to around

5.6 or lower and stay there. She has brought her fasting morning blood-sugar numbers to ideal levels (around 75–85).

Here are the three core strategies I've come to view as most effective in my practice: (1) managing stress triggers, (2) establishing healthy habits, and (3) incorporating stress-reducing practices into daily life.

These strategies put control and peace back in your hands, where they belong.

STRATEGY 1: MANAGE STRESS TRIGGERS

Many sources of stress are unavoidable. But some can be minimized. Working intentionally to identify and reduce exposure to triggers of stress, or at least to manage your relationship with them, can go a long way to supporting healthy stress levels and blood sugar.

Identify the physical components of your stress response

To find your big stress triggers, first identify how stress shows up in your body. This will help you know when you're stressed.

Every person has different physiological signs. Some people feel like their stomach is tied up in knots. Others experience racing hearts, or sweaty palms. Everybody's experience of stress is different—and valid.

Common ways stress makes itself known include:

Muscle tension or pain (especially in the neck, shoulders, head, and back), headaches, fatigue, an upset stomach, a racing or hard-pumping heart, shortness of breath, dizziness, difficulty concentrating, chest pain, exhaustion, or shaking.

These physical symptoms are often accompanied by worried, anxious, catastrophic, hopeless, or overwhelmed thoughts.

Check in with yourself regularly to determine your stress levels. Start right now. Do you feel any of the physiological signs of stress? Write them down.

Space out other check-ins about every 2–3 hours, such as when you wake up, when you get to the office, before and after lunch, at the end of the day, when you get home, and before bed. Keep a journal if you can. Try it for a week.

You may very likely forget to do these check-ins, especially if you're stressed. Consider setting gentle calendar reminders or alarms at regular intervals (say, every 2 or 3 hours). Use vibration or soothing sounds to avoid startling yourself.

Take your check-ins to the next level by measuring your blood sugar at the same time each day. With a CGM (continuous glucose monitor), this should be simple to do. It will show you any relationship between sources of stress, the feeling of stress in your body, and your blood sugar readings. You'll start to figure out the impact that different events and levels of stress have on your blood sugar. Don't be nervous about getting this information. Understanding is the first step to helping yourself move forward.

PRO TIP: STRETCH MULTIPLE TIMES A DAY

Most people naturally carry tension somewhere in their body, often in the muscles of the back, shoulders, and neck. Take a few minutes to stretch your problem areas a few times a day. Set a reminder if needed. It makes a difference.

Identify your stress triggers

When you feel the physical sensations of stress, trace the sensation back to a cause. There *is* a cause. Let's identify it.

It might be obvious (you have a deadline today). It might not be (constantly feeling unsafe, policed, or judged). If you can't identify a specific cause right then, try thinking about what might be affecting you subconsciously.

Everyone has different triggers. For example, one of my dear friends is a psychologist. Vulnerable conversations are her bread and butter. But she experiences the possibility of physical confrontation as very stressful. Another of my friends is a martial arts instructor. Physical confrontation is *her* bread and butter. Ask her about her feelings, however, and she feels very stressed.

We all respond to events differently because we've been through different things. That's okay! In fact, it's more than okay. Everybody's sources are a result of what they've experienced in their lives. Your body is just acting to protect you. Don't judge yourself based on a source or trigger of your stress response. Just note it and patiently explore what you can do to help yourself.

Stress strategies

Sometimes you can eliminate a trigger of stress. If you are stressed out by crowds, for example, you can avoid the subway at peak times. If you don't like someone on your team at work, you may be able to switch to another team.

Unfortunately, managing stress triggers isn't always simple. Sometimes getting rid of one gives rise to another. You could solve your subway problem, for example, by taking taxis, but that can be expensive and cause financial stress. If you don't see an immediate solution (or partial solution) right now, you may find one tomorrow, or next week. Be patient with yourself.

Other times, there's no way around a trigger. Maybe you've gotten divorced, lost a job, are moving, or someone in your family is sick. In each instance, be intentional and strategic. Think about ways to reduce the amount of stress it causes you. After divorce, for example, you could proactively seek emotional support. Or if you're caring for grandchildren, you could rearrange your schedule or step back from some of your other responsibilities. You may have to have hard conversations with spouses, partners, children, friends, colleagues. You may need to ask people for help or to step up with their own share of responsibilities.

To optimally manage certain triggers of stress, you may need to do emotional work. Try journaling; writing down your thoughts and feelings can help get them off your mind. Therapy can help you work through concerns with a professional, if you have access to it. Traumas can be a major source of stress. Be patient with yourself and seek help. Just talking to a partner or friend can make stress feel more manageable.

Boundaries

One major source of stress in today's world is the constant pressure to say yes to invitations, work, projects, and helping others. But you *must* first put on your own oxygen mask before helping others. That's not selfish—that's pragmatic. When you set boundaries, you empower yourself to help better later if you want to. You also model healthy boundary-setting for others. Saying no can be scary at first, but you can start small. Then, work your way up to bigger things.

Often, people who feel obliged to always say yes think they have to explain themselves. But the word *no* is a complete sentence. No. Use your best judgment deciding if an explanation is necessary. Try to be as objective about it as possible. This can be hard to do. Many people have been deeply influenced by examples set in their earlier lives. Ask yourself if you've been conditioned to always say yes. If you need to work on your boundary setting, work on it.

PRO TIP: JUST SAY NO, LIKE JOANNA

My patient Joanna says a major part of her healing has been in setting boundaries with her family. She said, "I've been a certain way pretty consistently most of my life"—a way that always prioritized other

people's interests first. But then she started saying "No, I'm not going to cook that anymore." She says she's "gotten a little pushback,
but we're getting there, thanks to finally figuring out the easiest, most
peaceful solution . . . just saying no, I'm not going to be doing that
anymore every single day."

Learning to put herself first has been a challenge because that's
not how she and her family have normally done things. Joanna was
always the reservoir that people drew strength from. In many ways,
they probably didn't even notice that she was making so many sacri-
fices. But she began to say no, and her family found a new balance.
The people who most relied on Joanna found new ways to take care of
their desires, errands, and needs.

Over the last thirty-plus years, I've learned the most remarkable
thing: Most of my patients are caregivers, in one way or another. Often, they are caring for their children or for their aging parents, but
not always. Sometimes they are military people, veterans, volunteers,
or otherwise active in their communities. People with type 2 and prediabetes are sleeping less, cooking less, exercising less, and just generally less able (or predisposed) to set aside time for themselves.

PRO TIP: RECOGNIZE THE COST AND CHANGE THE PATTERN, LIKE DINA

Dina cared for her mother and grandmother until they passed. She
tells me it was worth it, but the stress impacted her own health.

"I don't want my children to have to go through what I went
through. I would do it again, for my grandmother and mother. I would
do it again because I love them. I'm the oldest sibling, so I'm kind of

used to being the caregiver. But it takes a lot for me to do that. I realize there's a cost. I paid for that. I didn't concentrate on myself."

Now Dina is giving herself the attention she needs. This is helping her children in two ways: by reducing the likelihood they'll need to care for her as she ages, by leading a healthy lifestyle, and also by modeling healthy self-care for them.

Common modern stress triggers that deserve your "no, thanks"

One of the most common mistakes people make is letting themselves get sucked into drama. Maybe people are gossiping at work. Do you need that in your life? No. Or maybe you got sucked into a debate in the comments section of a Facebook post. Did you need to do that? No. Social media is one source of stress you can just turn off altogether. You might also consider changing the places you hang out, or the groups you participate in. Maybe reducing stress means having fewer phone calls with judgmental relatives.

Start by imagining from scratch what kind of social engagement is healthy for you. Then work toward engineering your habits in that direction. If this means only talking or responding to emails, texts, or calls at certain times of day, go for it. Set that boundary.

A similar mistake is letting yourself get caught up in the news.

Stay informed! But be strategic about (A) when you read the news—maybe not on your more difficult days, just before bedtime, or when you haven't slept well, and (B) where you get your news—some news sources are more matter-of-fact, or less sensationalist, than others, which makes a difference in how you feel after interacting with them.

STRATEGY 2: ESTABLISH HEALTHY HABITS

Healthy habits are the first line of defense against stress. They are like bumpers in a bowling alley. When stress strikes, if you have healthy habits in place, you'll more naturally stick by them, and you'll be less likely to be disrupted by the stressful event. You're going to bounce between the bumpers of your habits, but they'll keep you in your healthy lane.

The irony of stressful times is that they are when we are most tempted to drop healthy habits—yet it's when they are the most important. The most stressful things we go through are usually unanticipated: deaths of loved ones, losing a job, divorce, illness. We need as much nourishment and as many healthy practices as possible to get through these difficult, and unavoidable, times in life.

But it's very challenging to start healthy practices *after* something traumatic has happened. Protect yourself beforehand. Get the healthy habits in place. Make healthy habits second nature to you *first*, before the unexpected strikes.

Identify and change less healthy behaviors

How do you normally respond to stress?

Some common stress-related behaviors include:

Switching to less healthy foods, bingeing, snacking, scrolling on social media, staying up late, sleeping in late, procrastinating, withdrawing from loved ones, lashing out, stopping exercising, avoiding fun activities, and indulging more in vices such as drinking, smoking, gambling, or retail therapy.

Identify your own stress-related behaviors without judgment. Many of us never had an opportunity to establish healthy ways to relieve stress.

Try to simply notice—again, *without judging*—what good habits you feel inclined to drop, and what unhealthy habits you feel inclined to start, when stressed. Don't beat yourself up. Plenty of people snack, binge, scroll, etc. when they're stressed. When you notice yourself about to do them, stay curious and ask yourself if there's something else you can do instead.

It's likely taken years for things to get out of balance, and it will take some time to bring things back into equilibrium.

Honor your stress responses

Many are self-critical of their responses to stress. They judge themselves harshly for what they react to, and for how they react to it. But both what stresses you out and how you respond to it have been determined by many factors beyond your control. There are five major determinants of stress:

- **Genes** influence what you perceive as a threat and how your body responds to this threat, including how much and when cortisol and adrenaline are secreted.

- **Childhood environment.** Did you grow up in a one- or two-parent household? Lots of siblings, lots of noise? Was it chaotic, stressful, quiet, loud? Some people love hustle and bustle; it's soothing to them. Others prefer quiet and calm. Most people prefer one or the other and can have stress responses to too much or too little activity.

- **Physical environment.** Your home, neighborhood, and the part of the world you live in all make a difference. If your environment makes you feel unpleasant or uncomfortable, that can give you a constant, low-grade stress response. Sometimes, there can even be toxins causing stress and you don't know it, such as Concentrated Animal Feeding Operations (CAFOs), diesel fumes, manufacturing exhaust, toxic groundwater, corroded pipes, and noise pollution.

- **How safe you feel influences stress and blood sugar.**
  Maybe where you live feels very safe. Maybe it doesn't. Based
  on your history, you and the people around you could have
  very different feelings of safety in the same place. It's always
  valid.

- **The body remembers trauma.** Whether experienced in
  childhood or the recent past, the stronger or more powerful
  the experience, the more powerful your body's memory, and
  the more powerful the physical symptoms of stress. Please
  take the time you need to heal and seek out resources to help.

Be patient with yourself and your stress responses. You didn't
choose your lot in life. What you *can* do now is accept it so you can
move forward.

STRATEGY 3: INCORPORATE STRESS-REDUCING PRACTICES INTO DAILY LIFE

In Cortisol Nation, rest is often viewed as a luxury, even an indulgence,
or a guilty pleasure. Many people think that if they slow down, the
floor is going to drop out from under them. Patients often tell me that
when they find themselves with unexpected free time, they hesitate to
take advantage of it in a restful way. Some feel worried about what will
happen if they slow down. Others tell me they feel guilty when they try.

But rest and relaxation aren't *threats* to health and stability. They
are the opposite: *keys* to it.

Just as stress is a physical event with physical effects, so are rest and
relaxation. They turn off superhero mode and get you off the blood-
sugar roller coaster. They help you reduce inflammation and bring
your digestive, endocrine, and immune systems back online. They
help you repair damage. They are *physical processes* that you need for
your *physical health*.

I recommend incorporating two strategic kinds of practices into your daily life: breathing exercises and restorative activities.

Breathing exercises

First, help your body calm down and get off the blood-sugar roller coaster with brief, scientifically proven breathing or meditation exercises. When you slow down your breathing and heart rate, your body will take that as a cue to slow down everything else, too. These are quick and efficient wins.

This is my favorite. It's simple, easy to remember, and you can do it anywhere.

Pause. Place a hand over your belly.

Inhale deeply through your nose. To really convince your body to relax, breathe long and deep into the bottom of your lungs. Feel your diaphragm, the muscle beneath your lungs, expand. Let your belly expand forward. You should feel your hand move. Keep your shoulders down.

Count to at least four seconds as you inhale (one Mississippi, two Mississippi . . .).

Hold for four seconds.

Then release for as long as you can, for at least seven and up to ten seconds.

Repeat this as many times as needed. I like to do it ten times, which brings me to about three minutes in total.

There are many other patterns or varieties of breathing and meditative practices that can help you. A variety of smartphone apps provide additional methods and guidance. Such exercises can also be a part of daily prayer, yoga, or meditation routines.

In line for coffee? On the subway? At work? At the dinner table? In a location where you don't want your stress response to be obvious? You can be anywhere and do breathing exercises, discreetly and effectively.

Do these exercises whenever you start to feel stressed.

I also recommend integrating them into your daily life, even in moments of relative calm. This helps your body get more habituated to this calmer state. For my patients, 2–4 times a day seems to work best.

Restorative activities

Second, help your body calm down and get off the blood-sugar roller coaster by creating a counterweight to stress.

Have fun! Laugh! Play! Really chill out! *Actually relax!*

Positive feelings expand in the mind and the body like a balloon. They take up space, pushing out negative thoughts and feelings associated with stress. When you do activities that bring you joy or peace, you create a new physical state. It's a lighter one, a more buoyant one, and more tranquil.

It's important to distinguish between simply *feeling good now* and *feeling good after.* Feeling good now can be fleeting: a physical sensation, or "switching off" or "going numb." A lot of us get home after a long day and just turn on the TV—but does that help in the long run? Sometimes switching off is important. It's got its time and place. But the best tool for fighting stress is an activity that makes a real change to how you feel.

When you choose restorative activities, ask yourself: What makes me feel *better*, specifically, more peaceful, or more energized, when I'm *done*? What *restores* me? What helps me feel connected to others and the world? What gives me meaning, love, or joy? Don't necessarily focus on how you feel while you're doing it, but after.

Some ideas you could try are a warm bath, a soothing cup of tea, reading a book, dancing, going outside, listening to the birds, looking at butterflies, hanging out with your dog or cat, a massage, singing, walking, watching comedy, getting acupuncture, knitting, stretching, girls night or guys night, sexual activity and connection, playing music, yoga, volunteering in your community, exercising, or praying.

Activities that help you feel connected to other people might be especially powerful. Unfortunately, one of the first things that drops off our awareness when we're stressed is connectedness to other people. We can feel too wrapped up in our stress to make the time to connect. Connection is one of the most important things you can do to expand the feeling of peace in your brain.

Do at least one fun, happy, joyful, or peaceful activity a day. I recommend giving it at least an hour, if you can. This may seem like a lot. But it really matters.

PRO TIP: HUM

I love recommending humming favorite songs to my patients, especially if they don't have a full hour or block of time to reset. Just listening to music is good, but listening is passive. Humming is *active*, and activity is an even more powerful way to expand the feeling of peace in your spirit. It's like smiling when you feel sad or standing confidently when you feel self-conscious. Doing activities your body associates with positive emotions instead of passively consuming media has a stronger likelihood of boosting your mood. Humming, whistling, or singing your favorite tune is an easy gift to give yourself.

PRO TIP: BREAK A SWEAT

Exercise helps burn off cortisol, excess blood sugar, and other stress-related molecules such as adrenaline. If you know you're heading into a stressful period, try scheduling your exercise ahead of time. If you're surprised by a source of stress, see if you can squeeze in some physical activity. It may reduce the pressure and anxiety you feel around the stress. It may flood you with some feel-good chemicals that can help restore peace.

PRO TIP: LEARN TO PLAY, LIKE JANALEE

When I started working with Janalee, she realized that she had been raised to be a very serious, hardworking person. This wasn't a *bad* thing. But she had never made space for play. She decided to make a change. She decided to learn how to play.

"I've had to learn how to become more restful and take time and calm down," she told me. "I had a mother that lived that way," she said, referring to her mom always being so serious. "So I am trying to learn how to play. I was never taught as a child. I'm actually scheduling play time in my days off. Play for me right now is playing the piano. I bought a piano. I'm sitting down and playing the piano . . . or looking at a recipe book . . . or reading a book. Making the time to read hasn't happened before."

Janalee also uses a wearable technology device that gives physiological feedback. It tells her when she might want to take a break. She listens to the wearable technology device for insights and trends. When it gives her feedback that her body is in a state of stress, she plays the piano or reads.

Janalee tells me she's realizing more and more that play isn't lazy. It's *recovery*.

PROGRESS, NOT PERFECTION

Stress can seem like a tough nut to crack. Many factors are always at play, and the unexpected is always right around the corner.

But facing it head-on helps with health and well-being in countless ways. Stress is powerful and may be the key element of the Yates Protocol that you need to address to help manage and reverse your type 2 or prediabetes.

Always remember that change takes time. Big change happens through the course of a bunch of smaller changes. Give yourself some grace and don't beat yourself up for mistakes.

Remember: progress, not perfection.

In this chapter you learned:

- Stress is the most widespread cause of type 2 and prediabetes.

- When stressed, sugar is released into the blood, dragging you onto a blood-sugar roller coaster and contributing to type 2.

- Chronic stress negatively impacts the brain and impairs the ability to make health-conscious decisions.

- You can restore blood sugar balance and health by managing stress triggers, building healthy habits, and incorporating restorative practices into your daily life.

Quick wins/first steps:

- Set boundaries against drama and any needless sources of stress.

- Delegate or share responsibilities. Have any difficult conversations necessary to distribute any burdens that lie disproportionately on you.

- Be intentional about when you engage in news or social media. Put limits on it if it stresses you out.

- Put healthy habits in place so they become second nature and can help you when the unexpected strikes.

- If you get knocked off track, focus on what's most helpful and feasible for you. Add back the rest when feasible.

- When choosing what to do with your time, select activities that leave you feeling better *after*. Don't necessarily ask, What feels good now? Ask, What will make me feel better later?

- Incorporate 1–4 three-minute breathing exercises into every day.

- Play. Relax. Have fun. In Cortisol Nation, this is a genuine health need.

II

Implementation

CHAPTER 6

Mindset

Some Quick Motivation and Real Talk About Making Changes That Last

CHAPTER MAP

This small but crucial chapter provides key mindset
tips for blood sugar success.

Mindset is critical to long-term success. It's the foundation of all sustainable change. A healthy mindset enables you to make choices that support your health. Tweak some elements of your attitude or perspective and you will give yourself the best gift there is, health.

Here are some of the ideas or mindset shifts I've seen help my patients the most.

EVERYBODY CAN DO SOMETHING

Many of us think we're too busy, we don't have the money, we don't have the time, we don't have the resources. That's not true. Everybody can do something.

One of my patients with type 2 diabetes, Ruth, is in a very difficult situation. While in an assisted care center she had a bad fall and was then confined to a wheelchair. She hasn't walked in four months. She has no control over the food she's given. It's all highly processed and nutrient deficient. In our first Zoom call, we discussed her situation and her options. She can't stand or walk. We don't know when or if she'll be able to do that. She must do something else. We figured out her budget and found she could get fresh vegetables delivered to the home. She could get fresh salad greens that are washed, prepped, and ready to eat every week.

***Brainstorming about this one small change helped Ruth switch from dwelling on what she* couldn't *do to getting excited about what she* could.**

This was just one small change. But it helped her get curious: What else could she do? She's in a very difficult circumstance, but it's not hopeless. She started taking the reins and her health and happiness improved substantially.

What steps can you take, even small, to help manage your blood sugar and start supporting your healing?

YOU DESERVE TO BE WELL

You are not crazy. Lots of people with type 2 or prediabetes have been shamed by so many people in their lives, maybe even the ones who are supposed to be their allies, cheerleaders, and helpers. That can make you start to believe it's all your fault. You really should be shamed, blamed, or judged and accept the stigma that comes with the diagnosis.

Anyone who implies this is wrong. It's not your fault. You deserve to be well. (You'd deserve to be well even if it were your fault.) You deserve, and can restore, genuine wellness: from the ground up, in partnership with your body, naturally, sustainably. You deserve to and *can* reverse your type 2 or prediabetes. You can get free not just from the dangers of this disease but also all the gaslighting you're being subjected to because you have it.

You deserve health and real health care. Your experiences are real. Your symptoms are difficult. You don't fit a cookie-cutter mold. That doesn't mean you can't heal. All it means is your path to healing is unique. The care for your health must focus on healing *you*, one area of wellness at a time. If health care hasn't worked for you so far, it's only because it hasn't been genuine care for your unique situation. You can heal. You deserve it.

SELF-CARE IS CARING FOR YOURSELF

We live in a materialistic world, so we're encouraged to think self-care means buying that pair of shoes you've always wanted, or budgeting for a spa day. These things aren't bad. Treat yourself if you want to.

But real self-care starts with these questions: How do I *care* for myself? How do I support myself? How do I prioritize what will help me be healthy and feel good in the future?

It's not always glamorous.

Lunch helps you keep cravings and appetite on track so that you don't overeat and make poor decisions at night. This is self-care.

Brushing and flossing your teeth after dinner helps you keep your hand out of the cookie jar later. This is self-care.

Meal prepping on the weekends sets you up for success for the rest of the week. It saves you from stressing about what to eat every day. This is self-care.

Starting an exercise regimen that you can sustain is self-care.

Getting assessed for sleep apnea is self-care. Wearing a CPAP device is self-care.

The Yates Protocol: *All of it is self-care.*

I have designed 100 percent of the Yates Protocol to be *care*.

Self-care is like caring for anybody else in your circle: It can be fun, but sometimes it's not. I love caring for my children, but parenthood is not without its challenges. It's not always a picnic. Same goes for yourself. Sometimes self-care is just engaging the gritty details of your life. Sometimes it's denying yourself things you enjoy but that don't serve you: staying up late, falling down YouTube rabbit holes, nibbling on the M&Ms on the reception desk at work. You make changes because they're good for you. You do it because you care about yourself. You set yourself up for success.

Care is a verb. It's something you do, actively. Get curious about your current habits and put anything you do to care for yourself in a place of honor in your mind. Putting money toward a continuous glucose monitor (CGM) could be more important than almost anything else.

The fun thing about self-care is that the more you do it, the more natural it becomes. You heal yourself while you do it, and it all gets lighter, easier, less like a chore and more like a gift you give yourself. Self-care is like a muscle you flex. Over time, you stop dragging your feet about stuff that's good for you and start to get in the habit of looking for more opportunities to support your health. Start small. Keep going.

HEALING IS IN YOUR HANDS, AND THAT'S A GOOD THING

You are the person who calls the shots. This is great, because you're the one living in your body. You get to choose. You get to decide what you do, how you live your life, what you eat, if you will exercise, if you'll prioritize sleep, how often you test your blood sugar, what you'll do in response to blood sugar data, if you'll be loyal to your self-care. These things are all up to you.

Sometimes patients feel scared, but it's because they don't realize how smart they are. How much do you know about your body? It's probably a lot more than you realize. You live in it. You know what it likes and dislikes. How much do you know about how bodies work? In reading this book, you are currently empowering yourself with knowledge about that. You know so much about your body. You get to choose.

YOU AND YOUR BODY ARE IN THIS TOGETHER

When blood sugar numbers start running up, this is your body telling you that something is wrong. It's telling you it needs your help. It can give you the energy, vitality, and health that you envision for yourself . . . but you need to help it first.

Your body knows what it needs more than anybody or anything. It has the capacity to be well. Any damage it's weathered has gotten in the way. *It's not your fault this has happened.* We live in a world that profits off our poor health. We go to stressful jobs: This is not great for our health. We lose sleep to take care of people and responsibilities: This is not great for our health. We eat highly processed, ultra-refined food designed to make money for the people selling it: This is not great for our health. We lose our fitness because we are exhausted and hurting and stressed: This is not great for our health. It's not your fault you've been thrown into this climate designed to harm health.

To facilitate a partner relationship with your body, you might want to start a dialogue with it. Tell it you're excited and are doing your best to listen and care.

Sandra began to view her body and herself as partners. I asked Sandra if she had advice for anyone starting out on a journey managing their blood sugar. She said:

> *"Let your body know you want to help; let it know y'all are partners now . . . And forget the years! It doesn't matter how long it's been that you've been doing this or that. It doesn't matter how long you've been on the path going the opposite way. Your GPS now has you on the main road . . . Just stay on the main road."*

SELF-CARE ISN'T SELFISH

It's hard to find or to make the time to take care of yourself in today's world. But it's crucial: It's crucial for you, for your future, and for the people around you, too.

PUT HABITS IN PLACE BEFORE "LIFE STARTS LIFE-ING"

We are creatures of habit. Everything that comes naturally to you now is a habit. Habits can change. They don't change overnight. But they change. The way to change them is to keep facing forward with grace. The goal is progress, not perfection. You've got old habits you might not love, but if you keep facing forward with grace for yourself, you'll become less beholden to them and more habituated to the ones you like. Sometimes you won't even notice it's happening. But it will be.

The key to long-term health is building habits that you can keep up relatively easily. Get your healthy habits in place and you put yourself on a track to longer-term health, vitality, energy, flourishing—and it's not an uphill battle. It's not some Herculean task. It's just what you do every day.

When life starts getting crazy, the first thing people naturally want is the easy stuff. It's natural to be low on energy, willpower, and zest and therefore to be more inclined to reach for convenience and instant gratification. When life gets crazy, most people stop eating healthy food, exercising, and doing all their healthy stuff. Ironically, this is when it's most needed.

Healthy habits are guardrails, like the bumpers at bowling alleys. Life gets crazy, but if you've already meal prepped, if you've already got your gym bag packed and by the door, if you've got healthy foods frozen in your freezer, they're already there for you. Healthy habits help you stay in your lane.

Pam

Habits are tough to start but become strategic in your wellness journey. They become like an old friend, comforting and consistent messaging for you to love yourself for what you have accomplished.

Slowly build healthy habits into your life. Take them one at a time. Turn them into the easier stuff. Then, when life gets hard, the habits will help make it easier.

Give yourself the gift of putting healthy habits in place *now*, so you can stay healthy and sane *later*.

TAKE BABY STEPS

Sometimes jumping into an entirely new routine is great. It's a jump start. But other times it's just daunting. In that case, ease into new habits slowly. It's important to know yourself and what kind of change works for you. Most of the time, I see people succeed through implementing change slowly. Here are some options for how to do that:

- Choose one or a few small things to change each week: for example, unsweetened tea instead of soda, walking instead of taking the subway, or bringing your lunch to work. Once the small change you've made becomes natural to you, add another one.

- Break big goals into smaller goals. If you have a goal in mind, but it seems too big, break it down into smaller pieces. For example, instead of giving up sweetened beverages all at once, first reduce your intake to one sweetened beverage a day; dilute it to one-half water and pour the rest out. If you don't know where to start with healthy eating, try just adding greens to dinner. If you can't imagine exercising for 30 minutes every day, start with 10.

- Just try. Sometimes a change is scary, and a good way to make it less scary is to tell yourself you're just going to try it. Tell yourself you'll just try it once or twice, or for a few days, or for a week, or a month. Pick a time frame that feels reasonable. Then do it and evaluate how you feel. Chances are good you'll feel *better*, which will prove to you that it's worth it and will also give you some motivation to keep going.

For my patient Reverend Lorraine, the stress of getting diagnosed with type 2 triggered unhealthy snacking. She told me:

"When I learned about high blood sugar . . . I didn't know what to do about it. Other than be depressed. I was just bummed out for a very long time. And I think that may have even started me looking for chips and snacks and just whatever I could eat to kind of calm myself down."

She knew she couldn't keep that up—it would be bad for her physical and mental health.

How did she stop? She decided to give herself a month to process everything. She gave herself a month to just think about what she was learning about having type 2 and start incorporating new changes slowly.

She decided to improve her sleep hygiene first.

"I could tell a difference in how I felt in the morning when I did not entertain YouTube for two hours at night, all under the excuse of 'it's my downtime.'"

PROGRESS, NOT PERFECTION

The goal to set is: better. Progress. Building healthy habits into your life in sustainable and enjoyable ways. That's part of why you don't have to go full steam ahead on all five steps at once. Keep everything feasible for you. Heal yourself in the ways you most need to be healed. Keep repairing your metabolic machinery and keep bringing those numbers down.

Dina said to me:

> *"I've kept at it and it's working. When you're making effort, and you get results that it's working, you don't mind being consistent and continuing to work on it . . . And then, those mistakes that you make? It's like Dr. Yates says, don't beat yourself up. There's always tomorrow. It's the next meal. It's the next day. Keep going."*

We're all human. Perfection is unrealistic. You don't need to be on a slingshot to the lowest A1C in record time. That is too much and unsustainable. Just face forward, keep going. Stack one healthy habit onto another and focus on yourself and how you feel whenever life gets tough.

This healing journey is about progress, not perfection.

CHAPTER 7

Testing for Success

Identify Food Sensitivities, Keep Your Favorite Foods, and Heal with
These Proven Continuous Glucose Monitor Strategies

CHAPTER MAP

This chapter explains why testing is necessary
for blood sugar success and how to do it with a
continuous glucose monitor (CGM).

KEY SECTIONS

- Type 2 and prediabetes: the tests, numbers,
  and goals
- CGMs
- CGM tips
- Getting to the bottom of blood sugar spikes
  after meals

Edna sat across from me and looked down at her hands. She was tearing up a piece of tissue she had plucked out of the box I kept on my desk. Something was eating her up inside.

"How are you feeling?" I asked.

"I'm nervous," she responded. "Yeah. I'm afraid. It's fear, I think. I have a pretty big feeling of fear right now."

She told me it was because of her high blood-sugar numbers. She was in a pretty dangerous blood-sugar range. I had to agree with her on that. But that wasn't what scared her the most. She couldn't figure out what she was doing wrong. She'd found an eating plan online and gotten it okayed by her previous doctor. It was supposed to be helping. It was doing the opposite. She kept experiencing blood sugar spikes. When she went to bed, her levels were in the 200s, and her morning sugars weren't getting any better.

"Did I make a mistake I can't fix? Is there something wrong with me?" she asked. "I know type 2 is reversible . . . Why aren't my morning sugars coming down? Other people seem to be doing it. Have I gotten myself into a mess I can't get myself out of?"

First, I assured Edna there's nothing wrong with her and asked if she was testing her blood sugar.

"Sometimes!" She looked off to the side. "But I don't have a prescription for a CGM, and I don't always carry my glucometer and testing strips with me. When I do have the opportunity to test, I don't always do it because my fingertips are bruised and sore. I hate testing. It's way more painful than they make it out to be. And the test strips expire quickly and are expensive. Trying to keep up with blood sugar testing is a wild card for my budget."

I nodded. Edna was right. It is *way more painful than they make it out to be.*

I told her that we'd work together to find a way for her to get a CGM. This was step number one. It would provide her with nearly painless and convenient insight into her blood sugar spikes.

We'd use it to figure out what was going on in her body. There was an answer to what was dragging her blood sugar around. We'd unlock it with data.

Three months later, Edna and I sat down together again.

She just started chuckling. It was a laughter of relief. She sounded like a totally different person. I loved seeing the bright look of peace on her face. There was more levity in her smile and voice.

Just a week after starting to use a CGM, Edna had found her answer. She discovered that her body responded poorly to a few kinds of legumes that were major features of the eating plan she'd gotten okayed. These legumes are in the category of food that heals, but every person is different. They just weren't right for Edna's body at that time.

So, Edna removed them from her diet. She tried other kinds of legumes and found a few that worked great for her: no big blood sugar spikes! She also made sure to load every meal with leafy greens, protein, and healthy fat, as advised by the Protocol. She ate the protein and greens first.

Her numbers started improving: All her post-meal blood sugar numbers were in the range of 20–40, no more than 50 mg/dl, and her morning sugars began to slowly inch down. She was so relieved.

"Dr. Yates! I'm going to be okay!"

So many people come to me frustrated or anxious because something they'd been told would work for them isn't working. Maybe they were given a list of foods from their doctor, or they heard a podcast episode.

The first question I almost always ask is: "Are you testing your blood sugar?"

There's an answer to persistent blood sugar spikes. There's *always* an answer. It's in the blood sugar data.

Once you know what's happening in your body, you can address it. What gets measured can be improved.

INNATE WISDOM

Your body is the authority on what it needs. You can read all the books on type 2 and prediabetes in the world (including this one), but the truth is: No one will be able to tell you what heals or hurts your blood sugar levels better than you.

Even in my earliest years of practicing medicine, I noticed that foods that often work for most people still don't work for some. I've seen patients have blood sugar responses to *zucchini*.

Beyond moderate variations in blood sugar responses to foods, you can develop significant food sensitivities. In my practice I've seen a strong correlation between foods that show up for people on sensitivity assessments and foods that trigger blood sugar responses. Why? Food sensitivities create internal stress and inflammation, which can spike blood sugar. Studies are beginning to confirm the importance of bio-individual sensitivities to foods: Tailoring each person's diet to their unique gut microbiome status improves post-meal blood sugar numbers. Almost no one's talking about this. It's time to talk about individual blood sugar responses and food sensitivities so people have more clarity about what might be hijacking their blood sugar levels.

Dina

"What may work for one may be detrimental to someone else. Dr. Yates's program says: *This usually works*. But you need to test. Because it may not work for you. Half a banana? Some people can. I better not eat a banana, period! You don't know these things until you actually test."

IT'S NOT JUST FOOD

Sleep, exercise, meal timing, hydration, stress, physical environment, allergies, pain, medication, supplements, mood, caffeine, other health conditions . . . These all play a role in your blood sugar.

TWO SOURCES OF DATA

You can get information from your body in two ways. Start with your symptoms.

How do you feel? That's data. If you feel like you haven't slept well, you probably haven't. If you feel energized throughout the afternoon, you're doing something right! Fatigue, low mood, shakiness, a racing heart: These are possible signs of a blood sugar crash. Listen to all of this.

But data also comes from devices. Your individual blood-sugar data is how you compare strategies and see which work best. It's how you improve.

Trying to heal without data from a device is like getting in your car and driving with no directions. Without that data, you don't really know what you're doing. You also need these important numbers for your doctor and other health professionals to be able to guide you appropriately.

Get a testing device, hopefully a continuous glucose monitor (CGM). Learn how to use it. It will be your objective guide. It will remove confusion and anxiety about what you can eat and how to heal. It will put you back in control. It will help set you free from the frustrations and dangers of high blood sugar.

Pat

"A CGM can make you accountable. The proof is immediate: It shows how your body reacts to food. I had to stop making oatmeal for my breakfast because my blood sugar shot up so high. Once I got the CGM, it made a world of difference. I was in charge of my body, and food was now going to be my medicine!"

If you don't have a sensitivity to a certain food, you can probably find a portion, even if very small, that you can eat while keeping your blood sugar in a healthy range. Over time, as you learn how your blood sugar works, you can experiment and reintegrate small amounts of treat foods or desserts at special occasions without risking your health. Blood sugar testing is the only way to do this safely.

Remember, diabetes is an inflammatory disease. The higher your blood sugar levels are, and the longer they are elevated, the more this damages health. Blood sugar spikes slow down healing. Figure out which foods and lifestyle choices help you maintain the most stable blood-sugar levels and you accelerate healing and reversal of your type 2 or prediabetes.

BLOOD SUGAR MEASUREMENT DEVICES: GLUCOMETERS AND CONTINUOUS GLUCOSE MONITORS (CGMS)

There are two major kinds of testing devices you can use at home: glucometers and CGMs. Glucometers are the most popular and well-known devices: the ones where you prick your finger and put a drop of blood on a test strip. They were the only devices for years. But they can be painful to use, inconvenient, and provide less data than CGMs.

I strongly recommend obtaining a CGM because they are better devices and becoming more available, including via over-the-counter access in the US.

CGMS

CGMs are little biosensor monitors you attach to the back of your arm usually for 10–14 days at a time, though some up to 180 days. They provide 24-hour insight into your blood sugar levels. The technology for blood sugar level sensing devices continues to evolve.

You don't have to do anything to get your data other than change the sensor once every 14 days or according to your device's specific requirements. The CGM collects all the data for you and sends it right to your smartphone and/or your health-care provider (or others you select).

The quality of the data is the biggest win. CGMs are a little less precise than glucometers, but everything else about CGM data is a major win. CGMs provide powerful data that you can use to make the best decisions for yourself. You measure, you experiment, you improve. CGMs give you an opportunity to be your own hero.

Most CGMs have their own apps from the CGM device manufacturer that let you see your blood sugar responses to your lifestyle.

Specific apps also provide good data analysis tools and might let you input your meals, your sleep, your exercise, your moods, too. The most user-friendly apps let you take photos of what you eat and drink, and the software figures it out. Apps can help you identify what's working for you and what isn't, and some make recommendations you can try. Some CGM-based apps are up to speed on the latest science and account for diverse influences on blood sugar, including the too-often overlooked influences of poor sleep and stress.

A final benefit is that CGMs can notify you, or caregivers or loved ones, when blood sugar levels go too low or high. It's up to you whether you use the alerts. You get to program your own settings. If you are type 1 or hypoglycemic, low blood sugar alerts are lifesaving, and the low blood sugar alerts cannot be turned off, for your safety.

CGMs are typically more expensive and difficult to obtain than glucometers. In the US, they are difficult to get a prescription for if you are not prescribed insulin. But the expense or the trouble of fighting with health professionals or insurance companies is worth it. It is vital to persist in obtaining a CGM. This could be the greatest gift you give yourself on your healing journey. Be sure to get access to the tools you need to be successful on your healing journey and prioritize this in your budget.

SHORT-TERM IS BETTER THAN NO-TERM

If you are unable to get a prescription for a CGM, and the CGM price tag is daunting, consider budgeting for a short-term commitment.

The ideal is to commit to at least three months. More is great, but do what you can. Try committing to three. You can decide what to do about your blood sugar testing after that.

The amount of insight you can get in a short time can be a game changer. A few months with a CGM could give you enough insight into your blood sugar that you can then transition to a glucometer, getting readings a few times a day, or on a case-by-case basis, using the insights the CGM taught you.

If you can't commit to three months, try one month. To optimize the data you get, do a few days of business as usual, then start implementing the changes on the Protocol that you think are most strategic to make. As you make more changes with the Yates Protocol, you'll get quick feedback. You'll see what works and what doesn't. It's best to go longer than this if you can. Shop and ask around.

CGM TIPS

CGMs are very easy to use. Here are a few of my practical notes for patients.

- Read the information that comes with the CGM and its sensor. Check the manufacturer's website and product packaging info for tips and recommendations.

- Avoid doing sweaty things right before applying the new CGM so your skin is dry.

- Some people have reactions on their skin at the CGM location site due to the adhesive on the back of the CGM. Before applying the device, be sure to prep by washing your skin, drying it, and wiping it with alcohol.

- It can be a challenge to get the CGM to stay on the skin for the full length of time. You can buy protective "skins" or patches (they look like an oversize Band-Aid) to place over/ around it to help keep it in place longer.

- If you apply the new sensor before bedtime, be sure the warm-up time of the sensor is complete before you go to sleep; read the sensor recommendations.

- If you are a side sleeper and you put your CGM on the back of your arm, which is where most are supposed to go, make sure you know how you roll while you sleep so you don't roll over it. If you roll over it, you will get a low reading and trip an alarm, creating a middle-of-the-night false alarm. Be aware of that. Don't be paranoid, but the outer third or half of your arm may be a no-placement zone. Consider placing it more toward the inner part of your upper arm. You can get into bed and notice how you roll when you start to roll over from being asleep so that you see where to place the CGM on the back of your upper arm without rolling on it.

- You can wear the CGM to the gym. Just be careful not to snag it on your clothes or other materials, as this might loosen the sensor, knock it out of place, or break off the filament and make it stop working.

- CGMs are water-resistant, not waterproof. Wearing a CGM while sweating, exercising, and at the gym is okay. If you are swimming, please note: Most devices recommend that you keep the sensor underwater for less than 30 minutes. If you want to swim longer, be sure to wear the large waterproof bandage supplied with the CGM or purchased separately. Don't take the sensor deeper than three feet (approximately one meter). Always read the CGM device recommendations for use when swimming or in the ocean or other sustained wetness environment.

- Avoid exposure to salt water, seawater, or ocean water.

- Consider doing the first application with trusted health professionals at your doctor's office or at your pharmacy so you can gain familiarity and support when this is new to you.

- When you first start, go through your normal routines for a few days so you can discover how your starting habits impact your blood sugar levels. Get a baseline understanding so you can see the effect of changes. If you've started making changes before the CGM, go ahead and keep up with them once you start using it.

SHOULD YOU SET BLOOD SUGAR ALARMS? ALARMS VS. DAILY REVIEW

CGMs come with the option to set notification alarms when your blood sugar levels reach a certain high or a certain low. Whether you use this feature is up to you.

If your blood sugar levels often crash, and to dangerously low levels, such as below 70 mg/dl, then it may be important, even lifesaving, to set an alarm. This is always the case for people with type 1. If you have another form of hypoglycemia and blood sugar crashes, then it may be for you, too.

Do you want to intervene in your blood sugar before it rises to a certain point? If so and if alarms don't bother you, then you may wish to set a notification for certain blood-sugar highs. Then you can do some exercise. You can go for a walk around your block, up and down your street, or maybe just in your driveway. If you're at work, you can walk up and down the stairs or do some squats. If you are at home, you can do some push-ups, some squats, some wall sits. That can help keep your numbers from going up, up, up. If you frequently experience blood sugar crashes, this will also help them from plummeting back down.

Yet for many people, it's best not to set alarms. Freaking out can cause your stress hormone cortisol levels to spike and end up driving your blood sugar higher. It's important to know yourself. I'd rather you do a daily review at a time that is calm and stable when you can honestly reflect on what happened.

In fact, all people should do this daily review when you are calm and stable and can honestly reflect on what happened. Even those who get alerts.

TYPE 2 AND PREDIABETES: THE TESTS, NUMBERS, AND GOALS

Here are the basic numbers you need to know.

Blood sugar (blood glucose) measures the amount of sugar in your blood: It's provided in milligrams per deciliter (mg/dl).

Fasting morning blood sugar (fasting blood glucose) is a test of blood sugar after an 8- to 12-hour fast, typically in the morning. Fasting morning blood sugar is known by researchers as **fasting blood glucose**, though it also commonly goes by the name **fasting blood sugar**. Sometimes people call it their "morning sugars." I like to say "fasting morning blood sugar," so we are all on the same page.

Fasting morning blood sugar is a diagnostic tool.

Anything above 126 mg/dl is considered type 2 diabetes.

The range 100–125 is prediabetic.

The established healthy fasting blood glucose range is between 72 and 99 mg/dl.

My preferred ideal range is 75–95. The best control I've seen is when people awaken in the 80s. It's not about trying to get lower and lower. The body needs some sugar in the blood—just not too much. I don't want to see it under 70: That's hypoglycemia. You might feel dizzy, faint, or nauseated.

Ideally, you'll start seeing improvement in fasting morning blood sugars soon after you begin the Yates Protocol—within a few weeks.

Oral glucose tolerance test (OGTT) provides insight into your body's response to sugar. After a fast of 8–12 hours, you consume 75 grams of pure sugar dissolved in water. You measure your blood sugar one hour and two hours later. How much has it risen? If higher than 200, this signals diabetes. If between 140 and 200, that's technically prediabetes. This is a test most commonly done in a lab.

A1C (or hemoglobin A1C, or HbA1C) is the most common and currently authoritative diagnostic tool. It measures average blood sugar over the last three months.

When sugar enters your bloodstream, it attaches to hemoglobin, a protein that is a part of red blood cells. A1C measures what percentage of the hemoglobin of your red blood cells is coated in sugar. It's normal to have some sugar attached to hemoglobin. But too high signals there is too much sugar in your blood.

Type 2 diabetes is 6.5 percent and above.

Prediabetes is 5.7 to 6.4 percent.

If you start out type 2 and reduce your numbers to the prediabetic range, it is considered "remission."

Technically, 5.6 percent and below is "normal" or in the "healthy range."

If you start out with your numbers at 6.5 percent or higher, then get your numbers down to 5.6 percent or lower, this is considered "reversal."

An A1C of 5.6 percent is great, but an ideal A1C is 5.4 percent or lower: between 4.6 and 5.4 percent. For someone who has been in trouble, getting anywhere into this range is absolutely wonderful. Some people who are older or with specific vulnerabilities may not have the easiest time getting to the lowest ranges, down to 5.2, 5.1, 4.8 percent.

Passing over from prediabetic to type 2 diabetic is an emotional moment for a lot of people: full of worry and alarm. But it's a spectrum. The amount of damage from having an A1C of 6.5 percent is just about the same as 6.4 percent: It's 0.1 percent different. And 6.4 percent is 0.1 percent different from 6.3, and on and on. The damage isn't an on/off switch. The higher A1C is, the more at risk you are. That much is very clear. If your A1C is *anywhere* in the diabetic range—and even in the prediabetic range—you want to be bringing those numbers down.

A1C can be used to calculate average blood-sugar levels, measured in the standard mg/dl, with 7 percent corresponding to an average blood-sugar level of 154 mg/dl; 8 percent to 183; 9 percent to 212; 10 percent to 240. An average blood-sugar level that corresponds to the "healthy" level of 5.6 percent A1C or less is 114 mg/dl or less.

Post-meal (aka postprandial) blood sugar rise isn't a test used to diagnose type 2 or prediabetes, but it's an important tool. How much does your blood sugar rise after meals? Calculate the rise by subtracting your pre-meal blood sugar from your post-meal blood sugar. For example, if your pre-meal blood sugar is 120, and your post-meal blood sugar is 145, your post-meal blood sugar rise is 25.

How much your blood sugar rises after a meal depends both on your health and on what's in the meal. With diabetes, it is common to see a big spike after a meal, especially if it is blood sugar unfriendly—up by 60 points or more. A healthy body's response to a healthy meal exhibits a rise of 20–40 and no higher than 50 mg/dl after a meal, and it resets to where it was before the meal within an hour or two.

The goal for everybody is 20–40, as much as 50 mg/dl but no higher, after meals. For many people just starting out on this journey, 50 is a win. But the target for all is 20–40.

Typically, this is the first number you see improve when you begin the Yates Protocol, especially if you're focusing on nutrition. Blood sugar readings after meals are a result both of your metabolic health and of what you eat in that meal, so if you change what you're eating, you can see change here quickly. If your numbers are super high when you start, you may not see them quite this low at first. What you want to be sure to see is better than before. If you were previously seeing 100 point rises after meals, getting down to 60 or 70 is a win. You can't stop there. Keep going. Keep healing. Keep experimenting to bring those down. You want to see the 20–40, no more than 50, range soon after implementing the nutrition step.

If after a few weeks on the Yates Protocol your numbers are higher than this, either what you're eating is not agreeing with your metabolic machinery or you are responding in unusual ways to the food. If you're not implementing the nutrition step, it could be time to prioritize it. What is most likely to help you bring these numbers back down into a healthy range?

Speed of post-meal reset: You want to see your post-meal blood sugar numbers come back down to where you started within one, maybe two hours, of a meal.

C-peptide reveals how well your pancreas is working to produce insulin. It is a common measure of both type 1 and type 2 diabetes.

C-peptide is a by-product of insulin production. The pancreas produces nearly equal amounts of insulin and C-peptide, so if you make a lot of insulin, you will have elevated C-peptide. If you do not, you will have low levels of C-peptide.

C-peptide can be tested with the urine or fasting overnight with the blood.

A normal C-peptide result is 0.5 to 2.0 ng/ml (nanograms per milliliter). Low levels indicate type 1 or that you have type 2 advanced to the degree that the pancreas is no longer producing insulin. High levels of C-peptide might suggest insulin resistance, because when the body is insulin resistant, it typically overproduces insulin.

Finally, **fasting insulin** is often overlooked but is very important. It's a key indicator of how well your metabolic machinery works. High fasting-insulin levels suggest you are insulin resistant. It's a good test for *anyone* to get done regularly, even if seemingly in perfect health, especially if you have a family history of type 2. It's an excellent warning sign of metabolic damage and should be acted upon as soon as something begins seeming amiss.

Fasting insulin is also an important test for anyone who experiences hypoglycemia. Many hypoglycemic people are overlooked and not properly assessed or treated because they don't have sky-high blood sugar and A1C levels. Elevated fasting insulin is common for people who experience crashes.

To test fasting insulin, you fast for 8–12 hours, then take a blood test. Ideally, fasting insulin is less than 9 mIU/L (milli-international units per liter) and amazing if it's 5 or lower. If you are overweight or obese, fasting insulin levels might be higher, such as in the 13–19 range.

Your goal for yourself with all these numbers should be: improvement. Every measurement doesn't have to be lower than the last. The body operates with ebbs and flows. You want a better general trend.

Fasting morning blood sugar: Between 75 and 95.

This number depends on your numbers from the previous day, how well your metabolic machinery is working and healing, and how well you reset overnight. Ideally, you'll start seeing improvement soon after you begin the Yates Protocol, within a few weeks.

Post-meal blood sugar rise (aka postprandial blood sugar rise): The ideal rise after meals is 20–40, as much as 50 mg/dl but no higher.

Typically, this is the first number you see improve when you begin the Protocol, especially if you're focusing on nutrition. Blood sugar readings after meals are a result both of your metabolic health and of what you eat in that meal, so if you change what you're eating you can see change here quickly.

Once you start the Yates Protocol, you should start seeing numbers in this 25–40, no higher than 50 range. If your numbers are super high when you start, you may not see them quite this low at first. What you want to be sure to see is *better than before*. If you were previously seeing 100 point rises after meals, getting down to 60 or 70 is a win. But you can't stop there. Keep going. Keep healing. Keep experimenting to bring those down. You want to see the 20–40, no more than 50 range soon after implementing the nutrition step.

Speed of post-meal reset: You want to see your post-meal blood sugar numbers come back down to where you started within one, maybe two hours of a meal.

If it takes two hours, all is not lost. Your body has taken the meal in. Now you're processing it, digesting it; your microbiome and all the other things that affect your blood sugar are doing their parts in the dance. All the feedback is happening.

You definitely want to see it come down at least to the starting level, if not lower, before your next meal, which should be 4–5 hours later. The goal for people with type 2 and prediabetes is to keep resetting lower and lower. Help yourself get back down into those healthier ranges. This is why it's so important to refrain from snacking, to keep moving throughout the day, and to wait the full 4–5 hours before eating again. Give your body a chance to reset and you lift some of the burden off your metabolic machinery.

TTT: THINGS TAKE TIME

You can see some quick initial improvements, especially in your post-meal numbers. But full healing and reversal won't be a lightning switch overnight.

Your system took time to break. It likely took many years. It'll take time to heal. Most likely, it will be faster than the time it took for it to break. It'll still take time. Like most of the good things in life, it takes time.

TTT.

PROGRESS, NOT PERFECTION

Some people have the potential to completely reverse into the "normal" or "healthy" zones: fasting morning blood sugars between 75 and 95, A1C of 5.6 percent or lower. Others might get close. If you don't get all the way there, or your progress isn't lightning quick, congratulate yourself on progress and on getting your numbers down. This means less risk of serious illness or consequences. That's what we're really after here. Don't consider yourself a failure if your A1C doesn't become a 5.1 in three months. Bringing it down is a win.

If you see a stall, or numbers go up, maybe you've gotten out of touch with your healthy habits or aren't implementing the aspects of the Yates Protocol most important for you. Keep adjusting your life and habits to help you bring your numbers down bit by bit.

Progress, not perfection.

DON'T FEAR THE DATA

People are often terrified to get data. The fear is legitimate. They've spent much of their lives being blamed and shamed for their prediabetes or type 2. They've been told: *You're a failure. How did you let yourself get this way? How did you let this happen?* Looking at the numbers can feel like confirmation: *You let yourself get this way.*

False. You didn't *let* yourself get this way. No matter where you are with your blood sugar numbers, they're not a reflection of your worth. Data is a tool, nothing more.

The point of data is to help you know what's working and what isn't. Learn to be dispassionate. Don't measure self-worth one way or another. Numbers give you an objective sense of what's serving you and what isn't. This is a judgment-free zone. Measure so you can improve.

PRO TIP: KEEP CALM, KEEP GOING, LIKE SONIA

When Sonia first started the Yates Protocol, her numbers were high. She was confused and anxious about testing her blood sugar, because she thought she had been doing everything right.

"Looking at the numbers was a bit scary. When I pricked my finger and saw the number, I went into panic mode! What was the number? 400! I wouldn't have been upset if I had been doing something I knew was no good, if I'd had custard or white rice or something, but sometimes I had just eaten kale and quinoa! I thought to myself, okay, keep going. I just need more understanding."

Sonia was right. As she started using her CGM, she got the data she needed. She got her blood sugar under control. Even though it was scary to get the data at first, this ended up being the secret to her healing. It's what enabled her to remove the fear and regain balance and control.

PRO TIP: TRUST THE PROTOCOL AND BE ENCOURAGED, LIKE STAN

Stan started out in bad shape: A1C 10.0 percent, fasting morning blood sugars over 220. Like many, he came to me carrying some discouragement. All his prior experiences gave him low expectations for himself and his healing potential.

As we made changes, starting with nutrition, he started to see improvement. He felt really encouraged. His numbers kept going down and down. "Dr. Yates, this is wonderful!" he said. "You mean, I don't have to become a vegan or vegetarian or be perfect to bring my numbers down?"

"No. This is not required," I said.

Be encouraged. No matter where your numbers are, you can start bringing them down just about immediately. You might have sky-high numbers starting out, but this is okay; it's an opportunity to heal. The Yates Protocol works.

INTERPRETING DATA: LOOK FOR TRENDS AND DON'T JUDGE

Do not obsess on any one data point. It's not a reflection of your worth. The data point suggests something is working or not working. Also, bodies are complicated. Blood sugar fluctuations depend on so many different factors. Unless you're doing a specific experiment to see a specific effect of a specific food or exercise, just look for trends.

Reverend Lorraine started using a CGM and learned that her midafternoon snack, even though it was supposed to be blood sugar friendly, messed up her blood sugar levels before dinner and sometimes after dinner, impairing her sleep. She didn't know until she got the CGM that it was the snack causing this. When she figured it out, she just removed the snack. She didn't fall into a spiral of blaming herself. Now she eats more filling meals and doesn't snack. Her numbers are coming down. No shame, no blame, no spike!

SOME THINGS TO CONSIDER AS YOU REVIEW YOUR CGM DATA

If you are using insulin as part of your treatment, how does your blood sugar respond to your medication timing?

Did a particular food spike the blood sugar result?

Do feelings of stress cause high blood-sugar levels?

Does exercise affect your blood sugar levels?

Does vigorous exercise cause a significant rise in your blood sugar levels? How long does it take to come back down, and does it reset lower?

Does gentle exercise lower your blood sugar levels?

Did poor sleep happen because of high or low blood sugar?

If you awaken in the middle of the night with your heart racing and can't get back to sleep, does this track with a blood sugar low or a blood sugar high?

Does the "hangry" feeling happen at the same time as low blood sugar?

Does a late afternoon urge to snack happen at the same time as a high blood-sugar reading?

Does not drinking enough water, and being dehydrated, cause high blood-sugar levels?

Do feelings of anxiety or depression track with changes in blood sugar levels?

IDENTIFYING A PROBLEM

When you look at your CGM, what levels should concern you or pique your inner detective about what's dragging you on a blood sugar ride? The answer: anything that contradicts the trend of your progress.

Everybody on the Yates Protocol is at a different starting point. But everybody is seeing improvement. A red flag is when something happens that deviates from or contradicts the progress you're making. A red flag is when your levels are higher than what you've been seeing with your progress, especially with your morning blood sugars and your post-meal blood sugars.

For example, say you have made some changes in your nutrition, and you've started seeing post-meal rises of about 50 points. This is at the high end of the healthy range, but it's a big improvement over the 100-point rises you were seeing before the Yates Protocol. This is a win. If you have a meal and the rise is 80, that's something contradicting the trend. You've been improving. What happened to disrupt that trend? Get curious about that.

GETTING TO THE BOTTOM OF BLOOD SUGAR SPIKES AFTER MEALS

How do you make sense of a blood sugar response to a meal? Become a detective. There's always an answer.

Start with the basic question: Did you make the food at home? Did you know what was in it?

If you cooked at home and used something premade at the store, did you read the label? Do you know if there is added sugar? Things don't have to be sweet to have had sugar added.

Gravy, sauces, and salad dressings can all have added sugar. Read the labels. You'd be surprised what is hiding in there. Food companies get so clever. There are all those alternative names for sugar. Is it malted? That's a tricky name. (See page 34 for a list of clever sugar names.)

Is there breading on veggies or meats? Breading is usually processed carbs.

Is it ultra-processed or highly refined? These foods are problematic because they are nutrient poor. Plus, you could have a sensitivity to anything in them.

Be sure to check the serving size. Lots of sugar in a drink or meal can hide behind small serving sizes. For example, if the serving size says 4 ounces and the portion you usually consume is 16 ounces, you must multiply the listed sugar by 4 to get the real amount you are consuming. Beware.

Then, look at the carbs. Were they slow burning, complex, resistant starch kinds of carbs welcome on the Yates Protocol or did you eat any simple carbs? What was the portion? Two cups of white rice, a simple carb, or even of brown rice, a complex carb, will likely spike blood sugar. One cup could be too much for you. Portions matter.

Look at your beverages. If it's not water or unsweetened herbal tea, it could be the problem. If you're drinking anything processed, it's likely full of sugar. Supposedly "healthy" options purchased at stores, like bubble teas, coffee drinks, or green smoothies, can have hundreds of calories worth of sugar.

If it's a home-cooked meal and it's all Yates Protocol approved—it could be a food sensitivity triggering your spike. It's normal to have better responses to some foods than to others. You might be okay with white potatoes but not sweet potatoes, or vice versa; leaving the skin on might make a positive difference, too. Maybe you just need a smaller portion. Or maybe it's a serious sensitivity and you need to remove the food altogether, at least until you've made significant progress healing your gut and your gut's microbiome.

If you're still stumped and unsure what about a meal might have been the problem, you could try it a second time, especially if you know there were substantial extenuating factors such as stress, poor sleep, or it was after a big accident or upset in life. You can try again just to see if it happens one more time. If it does, then it's a problem with the meal for sure.

WHAT TO DO WHEN YOU'VE FOUND
A PROBLEM FOOD: SWAP IT

The amazing news is that there are always amazing swaps available. If you experience a response to white potatoes, try sweet potatoes with the skin on, or yams, cassava, rutabaga, beets. The options for root vegetables are endless. If it's lentils, try a different color lentil, or swap them for mixed beans, chickpeas, or quinoa. If it's white rice, try swapping it for wild rice, jasmine, basmati, or brown rice.

Sometimes, none of the swaps you'd like work, at least not in the portions you're hoping for. You might have major reactions to all varieties of potatoes, or all varieties of rice. Sometimes it doesn't matter how much skin you leave on a potato or whether the rice has the fiber jacket of its bran intact. You're still reacting. In that case you're going to want to look at a more dramatic swap, such as swapping rice for cauliflower rice ("rice" made from cauliflower), or grain-based noodles for zucchini "noodles." These are more nutritious than rice and grains anyway, so view it as a win.

If it really pains you to give up major favorites or it's a food that is deeply identified with your culture, and they're in the category of food that heals, know that it doesn't necessarily have to be forever. As you fix your blood sugar and reverse your type 2 or prediabetes, you absolutely cannot go wild and throw everything you've put into place out the window—but you will likely be able to experiment with reintroducing small portions of foods that are currently too much for your metabolic machinery to handle.

When reintroducing any foods, except on rare occasions, use the four groups I describe in chapter 1 as your guide.

KEEPING FAVORITES IS OKAY SO LONG AS YOU DON'T HAVE A SERIOUS FOOD SENSITIVITY

Noah first came to me with heart disease and congestive heart failure years ago. He recently returned with prediabetes. Putting this on top of the heart condition meant this was very serious. Even though he resisted at first, I convinced him it was a good idea to test his blood sugar response to meals. We started to see patterns. One was a reaction to large portions of white rice. He started reducing his portion to about half a cup and partnering it with protein, healthy fats, and lots of leafy greens. We got his blood sugar response to this meal into a healthy range.

Noah made sure his rice consumption didn't hinder his progress. He kept his portions low enough to have a healthy response to the meal and reset before his next meal. His fasting blood sugars and A1C are now showing steady progress, from being more than 6 now down to 5.5.

It's okay to want to keep your favorites. Blood sugar testing is amazing for this. If you don't seem to have a major food sensitivity to something, you can likely keep it by tweaking food combinations, cooking method, and portions to assure your blood sugar levels stay safe.

Never go above 50 mg/dl after a meal. Aim for 20–40. Do not incorporate any foods in any amounts that contradict your progress. Keep your responses in the healthy range to help you reset lower.

Keeping favorites: Make sure they're whole

To help you keep your favorites, first make sure that whatever food you're eating is in the most whole form possible. If you've been eating potatoes without the skin, for example, leave the skin on. If you're eating white rice or bread products, switch to whole grain.

You also want to be sure to cool your potatoes, rice, or grains before reheating them, which enriches their resistant starch content. That could help. If your blood sugar really went through the roof, cooling processes probably won't make up for the whole spike. But it can help your body minimize the response if you want to look for a way to keep eating this food.

Keeping favorites: Combine right

Start every meal with protein; animal protein is best if included in your diet. Eat fiber second. Plant protein usually contains carbohydrates, so if you eat a plant protein meal, be aware of this and experiment to find what's best for you. Dense plant protein sources such as lentils, chickpeas, soybeans (edamame), or tofu (soybean curd) may work well for this. If you're seeing your blood sugar spike in response to plant protein, try eating fiber (especially leafy greens) first, because fiber is a powerful blood sugar sponge.

Make sure you always pair any complex carbs/resistant starches with the other food groups and eat them last if you can.

Sometimes blood sugar control is a matter of adding one ingredient. When my family makes gluten-free waffles (page 196), we add ground flaxseeds. What a difference that makes! It also gives the waffles a rich nut-like flavor, and we avoid feeling like we're having a food coma after eating these waffles.

Try adding ground flaxseeds or greens to smoothies. Leafy greens, celery, cucumbers, or radishes make great additions to any salad, stir-fry, egg, or meat dish.

There are lots of practical affordable workarounds like these.

Keeping favorites: Portion experimentation

Noah's blood sugar couldn't handle 2 cups of white rice. But ½ cup, so long as it was with leafy greens and healthy fats, worked just fine. For some of my patients, rice is okay only at ¼ cup. That's quite a small portion, but it is what it is! As they heal more and reverse their type 2 or prediabetes, they will likely be able to tolerate some more.

If you experience a response to a food like rice, try cutting down to a quarter of the portion you'd normally consume. You want to see a blood sugar response that is 20 to 40, no more than 50 mg/dl, or in line with your current progress. If your blood sugar goes higher than this, reduce the portion even further or remove it entirely.

FOOD SENSITIVITIES

Sometimes you have a major food sensitivity, and that food spikes your blood sugar no matter the portion.

You want to avoid this food, at least for now. It's clearly disruptive to your blood sugar, which means it's almost surely disruptive to your gut microbiome and immune system, too. It's possible you could reintroduce it later after healing your gut's microbiome and the rest of your metabolic machinery. There are many other nourishing foods on the Yates Protocol, so no need to dwell on what you can't have.

TEST WITH THE OTHER STEPS IN MIND

You also want to keep steps other than nutrition in mind.

Meal timing could help with post-meal blood sugars. Many people tend to be more insulin sensitive and able to process blood sugar more efficiently earlier in the day. This is why I often say that if you're going to have fruit, with breakfast or lunch is ideal, and that it really is best to forgo dessert except on a special occasion. After a whole day of managing blood sugar, your body doesn't want an extra spike at the end.

Exercise can help, either before or after a meal. We are usually more insulin sensitive after exercise. You could also plan to exercise after a meal. But only use exercise to reduce the effect of eating certain foods occasionally, or not at all. You don't want to lose the healing benefit of exercise for the sake of a treat.

Stress and sleep always play a role. If you have a blood sugar response to a food or a meal and you don't know why, get curious about your sleep and stress. Data is best when you're comparing days with similar amounts of stress or sleep.

START SIMPLE, ESTABLISH BASELINES AND HOME BASES

Consistency can be a real gift. When you eat consistently, you get a clear picture of what works for you and doesn't.

Take your readings for a few weeks while implementing the healthy habits of the five steps and just start to understand. Establish a list of foods and practices you know are "safe" for your blood sugar. They're your friends. They're helping you heal.

Especially if you're particular or fussy, I really encourage you to eat as simply as possible in the early days. It'll make it much easier to home in on what actually works for you.

You can also always return to this home base if things get out of control. Learn the simple foods you know you can trust. Try to be here as much as you can. The more time you spend here, the easier it will be to figure out what causes unexpected spikes when they happen.

Then, you can experiment and adventure a little bit from this home base. To get the best insight into the effect of a specific food or activity, hold everything else as steady as possible. Scientists call this *controlling variables*. You want everything in your sleep, stress, daily habits, exercise, and meals to be as consistent as possible. You can intentionally introduce one new variable and see its effects. Noah and I kept his meal exactly the same but changed only the portion of rice. This showed the impact of the rice alone.

EXPERIMENT MOSTLY TO GAIN HEALTH

Many have an initial instinct, once they start seeing progress or establish a baseline, to go out and see how much they can get away with.

This is not the best attitude to have. I'm not saying it's wrong to want to experiment and to see where your limits are. It's okay to have a little bit of dessert or special occasion food here or there. But you don't want to always be pushing up against your limits, potentially damaging your body, as much as you think you can get away with. For optimal health, healing, and freedom, you want to focus on continuing to bring your numbers down and then keeping them there.

Don't get in the habit of asking *How much can I get away with?* Stay grounded in *What habits help heal me the best? What else can I improve?*

KEEP IT SIMPLE

Don't experiment, be adventurous, or try anything new if you're having a bad or off day. Try to stay in your home base. There's too much unpredictable happening in your body, and you're too sensitive—either physically, emotionally, or both—to handle a spike.

If you're in an unfamiliar environment or not cooking for yourself, be especially careful. You never know for sure what will be in a food prepared by somebody else.

Restaurants in particular can be a real problem. Their biggest interest is in making you enjoy their food, meaning they often put as much fat, salt, sugar, and additives in meals as they can. Sugars can hide in sauces, condiments, spice rubs, breading. You can request your sauces and dressings on the side, and you can also request that your protein and vegetables be cooked a particular way, such as steamed, grilled, or baked. But if you're unsure, err on the side of caution.

KEEP IT UP

Malika uses her CGM health data to make specific shifts and changes to her nutrition, meal timing, and exercise with the goal of getting her blood sugar levels consistently in a healthy range and keeping them there. She's found that adding fiber, focusing on breakfast and lunch, and working out in the morning are big wins for her blood sugar. She feels better *and* she has data from her CGM to prove that these changes are helping reset her blood sugar lower and heal. Yes! This is a way to win at healing blood sugar issues.

Now that the mystery around how these lifestyle elements affect Malika's blood sugar is solved, she continues to fine-tune her habits. She no longer has prediabetes, enjoys an A1C of 4.9, and continues to keep the healthy lifestyle in place, understanding that if she returns to what she was doing before using the CGM insights, the prediabetes and metabolic syndrome most likely will return.

Many health professionals consider the need for intentional management to pass once you've gotten your type 2 into remission and your A1C levels are in prediabetic ranges. They stop watching the blood sugar so closely. I agree that it's great you've brought the numbers down. But if you don't keep up the Yates Protocol, numbers can start rising again. When you get less vigilant or stop trying to improve, the metabolic machinery starts to degrade again.

All humans have different vulnerabilities. If you are vulnerable to becoming diabetic, you will remain vulnerable. You can regain health and functionality. But you must continue to guard it.

Fortunately, a CGM gives you the insights you need to stay in that healthy zone. You can keep an eye on your numbers. You can develop better metabolic flexibility and perhaps tolerate more variability in your eating with time, but stay vigilant. Keep collecting and responding to data. You'll be your own superhero, always.

In this chapter you learned:

- Every person's blood sugar response to foods, activities, and events is different. It is crucial to test your blood sugar, not to guess. What gets measured can get improved.

- There are two kinds of devices to measure blood sugar: glucometers and CGMs (continuous glucose monitors). CGMs are an amazing technology that provide 24/7 insight into your blood sugar.

- A1C is a measure of average blood sugar over the last three months. Technically, 6.5 percent or higher is diabetes; 5.7–6.4 percent is technically prediabetes. The goal is: *Better all the time.* You can get into *remission*, which is reversing from the diabetic range into the prediabetic range. But then you can keep going into *reversal*, down to the healthy range of 5.6 percent or below.

- Fasting morning blood sugar is an important metric. Technically, the healthy range is 70–99 mg/dl. I prefer a slightly tighter range of 75–95 mg/dl.

- The ideal blood sugar response to a meal is a rise of 20–40 and no more than 50 mg/dl.

- When experiencing spikes or seeing high blood-sugar test numbers, don't panic. Don't fear getting the data. Just stay curious. It's only data. It can only help you.

- Establish a baseline set of meals that are blood sugar friendly and you know work for your blood sugar. From here you can experiment with portions, other foods, or even occasional treats.

- Data is a gift. Use the ability to experiment to help support greater health, not to test and see how much you can get away with.

CHAPTER 8

Recipes

20 Easy & Delicious Recipes for Blood Sugar Success

GLUTEN-FREE · NUT-FREE · VEGAN

GLUTEN-FREE FLOUR

Makes about 7 cups • Active prep time: 5 minutes • Total time: 5 minutes

We have been a gluten-free household for over twenty years and developed this flour combination to support no-hassle gluten-free baking. This gluten-free flour mix is easy to make and will measure one-for-one with all-purpose flour. We make it in large batches so that cakes, biscuits, pancakes, and waffles are a snap.

For recipes that call for whole-wheat flour, the Gluten-Free Flour can be combined with ground flaxseeds (see tip for whole wheat substitute).

....

24 ounces brown-rice flour   16 ounces tapioca flour
16 ounces sweet-rice flour   1½ teaspoons powdered xanthan gum

....

1. Place all the ingredients in a large (4-quart) bowl.
2. Use a wire whisk to gently but thoroughly combine all the ingredients.
3. Store in an airtight container at cool room temperature away from direct sunlight for up to six months.

NOTES/TIPS: Brown-rice flour and xanthan gum can be found in many supermarkets and in health-oriented grocers. Sweet-rice flour and tapioca flour can be found in many Asian stores or ordered online.

The flour quantities called for in this recipe match the typical packages sizes. This way you can just pour the entire contents of the packages into your mixing bowl! Don't worry if the actual amounts contained in the packages are off by 1 or 2 ounces (such as 14 ounces instead of 16).

SUBSTITUTE FOR WHOLE-WHEAT FLOUR: When making a recipe that calls for whole wheat, use this Gluten-Free Flour recipe but replace one-third of the measured amount with ground flaxseeds. So if the recipe calls for 3 cups of whole-wheat flour, use 2 cups of this Gluten-Free Flour and 1 cup of ground flaxseeds. This helps to lessen the blood sugar impact. Test, don't guess, to see if this works for your blood sugar needs.

SIMPLE BISCUITS

Makes 10 to 12 biscuits • Active prep time: 10 minutes • Total time: 30 minutes

This is a combo-recipe for people looking for something yummy as a morning option. The gluten-free alternative has substantial fiber and less impact on blood sugar—a vegan option is included too. Of course these, and all refined carbohydrates, should be consumed in moderation (or not at all, depending on what your body will tolerate).

1⅓ cups whole-wheat flour
⅔ cup ground flaxseeds
1 tablespoon baking powder

Dash of ground nutmeg
1 stick (½ cup) butter, softened
1 cup milk or milk substitute

1. Preheat the oven to 375°F.
2. Put the flour, ground flaxseeds, baking powder, and nutmeg into a medium (2-quart) bowl. Use a wire whisk to gently mix these dry ingredients.
3. Use a fork to cut the softened butter into the flour mixture. Mix to an even consistency (it should look like sand).
4. Stir in the milk, a little at a time, until the mixture is stiff and clumps into a ball.
5. Use a tablespoon or soup spoon to scoop balls of the dough and place them directly onto an ungreased baking sheet, about 2 inches apart. You should be able to get 12 to 15 dough balls onto one sheet.
6. Bake for 15 minutes, or until the biscuits are golden brown on top.
7. Serve warm with your favorite spreads!

NOTES/TIPS: The biscuit dough can be mixed ahead of time, then rolled into a cylinder about 2 inches in diameter, wrapped in plastic wrap, and refrigerated. When ready to bake, remove the plastic, and slice the cold dough into approximately ½-inch-thick rounds and place directly on a baking sheet, ready for the oven.

MAKE IT GLUTEN-FREE: Replace the whole-wheat flour with the whole-wheat variant of the Gluten-Free Flour mix (page 194)

MAKE IT VEGAN: Substitute a vegan "butter" and oat or almond milk for the milk.

HERB AND LEMON SURPRISE: For a fun change-up, mix 2 teaspoons of fennel seeds and 1 teaspoon of lemon zest into the flour before blending in the butter.

GLUTEN-FREE · NUT-FREE · VEGETARIAN · VEGAN OPTION

GLUTEN-FREE WAFFLES

Serves 4 • Active prep time: 10 minutes • Total time: 20 minutes

This gluten-free take on waffles has substantial fiber and less impact on blood sugar. Of course these, and all refined carbohydrates, should be consumed in moderation (or not at all, depending on what your body will tolerate).

1⅓ cups Gluten-Free Flour (page 194)
⅔ cup ground flaxseeds
1 tablespoon baking powder
Dash of ground nutmeg
1 stick (½ cup) butter, melted
2 large eggs
1¾ cups milk or milk substitute, plus
   more if needed

½ teaspoon vanilla extract
¼ teaspoon lemon extract

1. Preheat a waffle iron.

2. Put the flour, ground flaxseeds, baking powder, and nutmeg into a medium (2-quart) bowl. Use a wire whisk to gently mix these dry ingredients.

3. Add the melted butter and use a fork to stir it into the flour mixture. The mixture will be lumpy but should have an even consistency.

4. Crack the eggs into a small bowl or measuring pitcher. Beat lightly with a fork or whisk. Add the milk, vanilla extract, and lemon extract. Mix thoroughly.

5. Add the milk and egg mixture to the flour mixture and stir until well blended. The batter will be thick but should be "pourable." Add a little milk if the batter is too thick. Do this a little at a time; if you add too much milk, the waffles will come out flat and thin.

6. Use a large mixing spoon or a ½-cup measuring cup or ladle to load the waffle iron. Cook the waffles as normal.

7. Serve warm with butter, a small amount of real maple syrup (like a tablespoon), or your favorite spreads!

MAKE IT VEGAN: Substitute a vegan "butter," and oat or almond milk for the milk.

ONE-POT MEAL · GLUTEN-FREE · VEGETARIAN · VEGAN OPTION

QUICK AND EASY LENTILS

Serves 6 as a main dish • Active prep time: 20 minutes • Total time: 35 minutes

This is a simple but hearty dish that can be enjoyed by almost everyone. It can go from cabinet to table in less than 45 minutes and is a reliable go-to for impromptu get-togethers or a quick and tasty main dish. Lentils are available in many varieties, and this recipe works for all. (See notes for pink or red lentils, which cook faster.)

A key to capturing the rich flavors of this dish is the finishing ghee that adds both flavor and mouthfeel to the dish. This starts with a base of ghee (clarified butter) to which potent spices are added.

FOR LENTIL BASE

3 cups lentils (brown, green, beluga, or French)

6 garlic cloves, peeled and very coarsely chopped

2 bay leaves

6 slices of fresh ginger root (cut fresh root into rounds about ⅛ inch thick and 1 inch in diameter)

2 cinnamon sticks

8 to 10 pods of green cardamom (optional)

1 tablespoon turmeric powder

5 slices of fresh lemon

¾ teaspoon salt

½ teaspoon black pepper

FOR FINISHING GHEE

1½ tablespoons ghee

1 teaspoon whole cumin seeds

½ teaspoon asafetida

½ teaspoon chipotle chili flakes (optional)

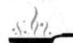

1. Put the dry lentils, ginger root, chopped garlic, bay leaves, cinnamon sticks, cardamom pods (optional), and turmeric into a 4-quart pot.

2. Add 8 cups (2 quarts) of water to the pot. Set to boil.

3. While the pot is heating, cut the lemon rounds and remove as many seeds as you can. Set aside.

4. About 20 minutes after the pot starts to boil, check the lentils for tenderness. Different lentils will reach tenderness at slightly differing times (between 20 and 27 minutes for most). They are tender if you are able to easily mash a lentil with the back of a spoon.

5. When tender, add the lemon slices, salt, and black pepper. Immediately start on the finishing ghee. Let cook for 5 more minutes, then turn off the heat.

6. To make the finishing ghee (during those 5 minutes): Place the ghee in a small skillet over high heat.

7. When the ghee is thoroughly melted and hot, put in the cumin seeds. Monitor the skillet until the seeds turn very dark (but before they start to smoke and burn!).

8. Quickly add the asafetida and chipotle flakes, if using. The blend of spices and high heat will be pungent.

9. Quickly add the hot ghee with its spices into the pot of cooked lentils. It will sizzle up. Stir it in.

10. Serve the lentils hot with rice or vegetables.

NOTES/TIPS: Ghee is available at most grocers, and asafetida can be found at many East Indian or Asian markets or purchased online.

MAKE IT FAST!: If pressed for time, this recipe can be accelerated by substituting split red lentils (masoor dal) and boiling the water before adding it to the pot (in an electric kettle or similar). With these changes, the cooking time for the lentils drops to 10 to 12 minutes. All other steps are the same.

VEGAN OPTION: Substitute a high-temperature vegetable oil for the ghee. Coconut oil or palm oil are good options.

DAIRY-FREE · NUT-FREE · VEGAN · GLUTEN-FREE OPTION

CONFETTI KALE

Serves 4 as a side dish • Active prep time: 20 minutes • Total time: 20 minutes

This is a fun and simple dish that is a tasty, high-fiber, healthy addition to any meal. Our family often makes this for breakfast in combination with turkey bacon and fresh-cooked eggs. We call it confetti kale because when the kale is chopped, it looks very much like strips of crepe-paper confetti. The festive vibe is reinforced by the pop of color added by the red peppers. Using a well-seasoned pan, these greens can be cooked with a minimum of oil for a calorie-friendly delight.

2 bunches of lacinato ("dino") kale
1 tablespoon olive or canola oil
3 medium garlic cloves, chopped

1 red or green bell pepper, chopped
1 medium onion, chopped
1 tablespoon soy sauce

1. Rinse the kale. On a cutting board, use a sharp knife to cut the leaves across the stems into strips about ⅛ inch wide. You can stack and cut about 6 leaves at a time. Put the cut greens into a clean bowl and set aside.

2. Heat the oil in a 10-inch (preferably cast-iron) skillet. When hot, add the chopped garlic.

3. Once the garlic is lightly toasted, add the chopped bell pepper first, and then the chopped onions. Sauté for about 1 minute.

4. Add the shredded kale to the pan. Let sizzle for 2 minutes. Then stir to combine with the peppers and onions. If it looks dry or starts to smoke, add up to 3 tablespoons of water, 1 tablespoon at a time. Don't make it too wet.

5. Add the soy sauce. Cover and let steam until the kale strips are limp and tender, about 5 minutes. Stir and turn off the heat.

6. Plate and serve.

MAKE IT GLUTEN-FREE: Replace the soy sauce with gluten-free tamari.

MAKE IT HERBY OR SPICY:

1 serrano or other spicy pepper, chopped	1 teaspoon fresh rosemary, chopped
	½ bunch of fresh basil, chopped

Toss your favorite selection or combination of pepper or herbs into the pan with the chopped garlic.

GLUTEN-FREE · NUT-FREE · VEGETARIAN · DAIRY-FREE OPTION

SWEET POTATO (YAM) CUSTARD

Serves 10 as dessert • Active prep time: 30 minutes • Total time: 75 minutes

This dessert dish is always a favorite. The mix can be used to fill prebaked pie shells, individual custard dishes, or as a plain and simple panful of goodness. Note that the orange-colored tubers that many folks (including me) call sweet

potatoes are really yams and are sometimes labeled as "jewel yams" in grocery stores. These are preferable to both "garnet yams" and white sweet potatoes. Orange juice is a family secret, and it really adds a nice flavor to the finished dish.

6 firm jewel yams (orange-colored sweet potatoes)
1 stick (8 tablespoons) ½ cup butter
1 cup packed light brown sugar
2 tablespoons unsulfured molasses
½ cup soy milk or orange juice

4 large eggs, lightly beaten
1 teaspoon vanilla extract
1 teaspoon lemon extract (optional)
½ teaspoon ground cinnamon
¾ teaspoon ground nutmeg
¼ teaspoon ground cloves

Peel, cut, and cook

1. Peel the yams. Cut into ¾-inch-thick rounds.
2. Place the yams in a 6-quart pot and add water to just cover.
3. Cover, bring to a simmer, and simmer until tender (about 20 minutes).
4. Use a colander to immediately drain (while hot).

Mix and mash

1. Preheat the oven to 375°F.
2. Place the warm cooked yams in a large mixing bowl. Add the butter. Use a potato masher to mash the potatoes while mixing in the butter.
3. Add the brown sugar and molasses. Mix well using a spoon or spatula.
4. Add the soy milk or orange juice. Mix well. If the mixture is still hot, allow it to cool until comfortable to the touch.
5. Blend in the beaten eggs.
6. Add the vanilla extract, lemon extract, if using, cinnamon, nutmeg, and cloves. Mix thoroughly.

Fill and bake

1. Transfer the mixture to a 9 by 13-inch baking dish or 10 individual 8-ounce custard dishes.
2. Bake for 40 minutes, until the top is slightly brown and the filling is firm. Serve warm or cool, but not hot.

MAKE IT TROPICAL ISLAND: Use a 6-ounce can of crushed pineapple with its juice instead of the soy milk or orange juice. Serious enthusiasts can substitute a similar weight of purple (ube or Okinawan) yams for the jewel yams.

MAKE IT AS PIES:

  Two 9-inch pie shells

Preheat the oven BEFORE you peel the yams. While the yams are boiling, prebake the pie shells. Most pie shells need to bake for about 15 minutes to get golden brown.

   Put the mixture into the prebaked pie shells instead of baking dishes. Use a dry toothpick to test for doneness; it should come out clean when poked into the center of the hot baked pie.

MAKE IT DAIRY-FREE: Substitute a nondairy butter for the butter, and be sure to check that the pie shells are nondairy, if using.

ONE-POT MEAL · GLUTEN-FREE · VEGAN · MEAT OPTION

HEARTY BLACK-EYED PEAS

Serves 6 as a side or main dish • Active prep time: 40 minutes • Total time: 90 minutes

This variation on the traditional African American dish eliminates the pork and incorporates just a touch of South Asian flavor. Turmeric adds flavor and color and is an excellent anti-inflammatory for those occasional aches and pains. Many ingredients overlap those used to make the Long Life Collard Greens (page 204), and preparing both dishes at once will save you some time overall.

3 cups dried black-eyed peas	1 teaspoon chopped rosemary
3 tablespoons olive oil	3 garlic cloves, chopped
2 bay leaves	1 medium onion, chopped
2 teaspoons fennel seeds	1 cup chopped celery (2 to 3 stalks)

1 jalapeño pepper, chopped (optional)   2 teaspoons ground turmeric
½ teaspoon sea salt   2 cinnamon sticks (optional)

Prep work the night before

1. Rinse the black-eyed peas in tap water. Place in a large (4-quart) bowl and add 2 quarts of water. They will need to soak for at least 6 hours. If you are not able to cook the beans before 12 hours have passed, change the water and refrigerate (this will prevent fermentation). In all cases, cook within 48 hours of soaking.

Cooking the black-eyed peas

1. Use a colander to drain the black-eyed peas. Rinse them in tap water and allow them to drain again.
2. Heat the olive oil in a 6-quart pot over high heat. Do not let the oil smoke or burn.
3. Add the bay leaves, fennel seeds, rosemary, and garlic. Sauté for about 1 minute.
4. Add the onion, celery, and jalapeño (optional). Sauté until the onions are limp (about 4 minutes). Stir to prevent burning.
5. With the heat still on high, add the beans. Stir thoroughly, then quickly add about 4 cups of water (until the beans are just covered).
6. Bring the pot to a boil, then add salt, turmeric, and cinnamon sticks (optional). Stir, cover, and lower the heat. Simmer, stirring occasionally, for 45 minutes (until the beans are tender).

MAKE IT MEATY:

About 1 cup chopped smoked turkey thigh

If you feel you absolutely must have that smoky, meaty flavor, chop up half a smoked turkey thigh and add to the pot right after the beans. A whole thigh would overpower the dish.

ONE-POT MEAL · GLUTEN-FREE · NUT-FREE · VEGAN · MEAT OPTION

LONG LIFE COLLARD GREENS

Serves 6 as a side dish • Active prep time: 30 minutes • Total time: 90 minutes

This is a variant of our family recipe for the wonderful greens that my mother and grandmother prepared for me. The traditional preparation has been modified to eliminate animal fats (particularly pork) and to enhance the flavoring with some unconventional spices. Many ingredients are the same as those used in the Hearty Black-Eyed Peas recipe (page 202), so preparing both at once will save you time overall.

---

3 bunches of fresh, good-looking collard greens (about 15 to 20 leaves)
3 tablespoons olive oil
2 bay leaves
1 teaspoon chopped rosemary
½ teaspoon ground cumin (optional)

3 garlic cloves, chopped
1 jalapeño pepper, chopped (optional)
1 medium onion, chopped
1 small leek (or half of a large leek), chopped
½ teaspoon sea salt

Chopping the greens

1. Trim approximately 1 inch from the bottom of the stalks of each collard leaf. Wash each leaf in tap water. Shake off excess water and lay flat on a cutting board.

2. Stack four to five leaves together alternately aligning the central stalks in opposite directions (first leaf oriented left to right, second on top right to left, and so on).

3. Roll the stack of leaves around their stems (it should look sort of like a green cigar). Hold the roll firmly and cross-cut at approximately every ¾ inch so that the roll falls into "rounds" of green strips.

4. Cross-cut the rounds so that the leaves are chopped into about 1-inch rectangles.

5. Repeat until all the greens are cut up. Set aside in a bowl.

Cooking

1. In an 8-quart pot, heat the olive oil over high heat. Do not let the oil smoke.
2. Add the bay leaves, rosemary, cumin, garlic, and jalapeño (optional). Sauté for about 1 minute.
3. Add the chopped onion and leek. Sauté until the onion is limp (about 2 minutes).
4. With the heat still on high, add a handful of chopped greens. Stir. Wait 1 minute, then add another handful. Continue until a little more than half the greens are in the pot. It may get hard to stir toward the end.
5. Add 1 cup of water and the sea salt. Cover and wait 3 minutes while the greens in the pot wilt down. You should then be able to easily add the rest of the greens without overflowing the pot.
6. Once all the greens are in the pot, add 2 more cups of water and stir well.
7. Bring the pot to a boil. Cover, turn the heat down, and simmer for 1 hour, stirring occasionally.

MAKE IT MEATY:

About 1 cup chopped smoked turkey thigh

If you feel you absolutely must have that smoky, meaty flavor, chop up half a smoked turkey thigh and add it to the pot right after the greens. A whole thigh would overpower the dish.

ONE-PAN MEAL · DAIRY-FREE · GLUTEN-FREE · NUT-FREE

UNFRIED CHICKEN

Serves 6–8 as a main dish • Active prep time: 15 minutes • Total time: 60 minutes

This "one-pan" main dish is savory, simple, and satisfying. It is a great option for those busy days when you want a tasty and hot meal but don't want to spend a lot of time making it or cleaning up. With this cooking method the chicken comes out crispy and hot, like traditional fried chicken, but most of the chicken fat stays in the baking tray instead of going into your digestive tract.

Try the basic recipe if you want to keep it simple and certain. As you repeat the recipe, experiment and be creative in your seasonings until you hit the combo that most tickles your fancy (see the variations).

. . . .

8 chicken thighs, skin on and bone-in

SUGGESTED SEASONING QUANTITIES, OR TO TASTE

1 tablespoon garlic granules (packaged spice)	1 teaspoon ground black pepper
1 teaspoon salt	1 teaspoon dried oregano

. . . .

1. Preheat the oven to 425°F.
2. Lightly rinse the chicken thighs. Pat dry with clean paper towels. (Immediately dispose of those towels.)
3. In a 9 by 13-inch baking tray, lay the chicken thighs out, skin side DOWN. Leave as much space as possible between the pieces (it will probably be pretty tight).
4. Season the chicken to taste by sprinkling the garlic, salt, pepper, and oregano on the exposed side of the 8 thighs.
5. Turn each thigh over so that all are now skin side UP in the pan. Repeat the seasoning on skin side.
6. Put the tray and its contents on the upper rack of the hot oven. Bake for 55 minutes. The skin will get crisp and take on a caramel color.
7. Remove the tray from the oven. Let the thighs rest for 5 minutes, then transfer them from the tray to a serving plate or platter (they will be hot, so use tongs or a fork).
8. Cleanup tip: While the rendered chicken fat in the bottom of the pan is still hot and liquid, lay 4 or 5 paper towels flat directly onto the oil. They will absorb the hot fat, and when cool they are easily scooped up with fresh paper towels and disposed of, without getting your hands messy or dealing with congealed fat in the sink.

NOTES/TIPS: This dish can be prepped ahead of time and refrigerated before cooking. Prep and season the chicken, then cover the tray with plastic wrap and refrigerate. Be sure to remove the plastic before baking. Put the cold tray in the oven before preheating so that it warms up with the oven. Cooking time starts when the oven reaches the specified temperature.

SPICE IT UP: Some additional spices to try (one at a time or in combination):

1 tablespoon ground cumin   1 tablespoon ground cardamom
1 tablespoon ground coriander   1 teaspoon harissa

Other spice combinations can be delightful; use your preferred spice combinations here. The amount of spice in this recipe is light. If you enjoy more flavorful food, please feel free to increase the amount of spices added, by double or triple.

ADD VEGGIES FOR A FULL MEAL: Once the chicken is in the oven, slice up a total of about 4 cups of any combination of your favorite vegetables—such as carrots, broccoli, asparagus, cabbage, or fennel bulb. Lightly toss these in a large bowl with 1 tablespoon of olive oil, ½ teaspoon of salt, and (if desired) a light sprinkling of any of the spices I've suggested. Turn these out into a different baking tray. Put the tray in the oven on the middle rack and bake for 20 minutes. Pull out with the chicken and serve!

ONE-PAN MEAL · DAIRY-FREE · NUT-FREE · GLUTEN-FREE OPTION · LOW-COST OPTION

OVEN-SEARED SALMON (OR BLACK COD)

Serves 4 as a main dish • Active prep time: 20 minutes • Total time: 50 minutes

This is a festive family favorite for holiday or "special occasion" meals with neither the dietary impact of ham or roast beef nor the cooking time and complexity of turkey. It can be prepared in less than an hour but still delivers a "wow" factor.

When making it, our family usually uses a full "side" of a king salmon (about

4 or 5 pounds), which delivers 10 to 12 servings, often with leftovers. That's a bit much in both volume and expense for everyday cooking, so this version is scaled down for everyday meals or smaller gatherings. For a cost-conscious option, see the variation using black cod (sablefish) instead of salmon.

. . . .

1 large bunch of lacinato ("dino") kale
1 leek or ½ large onion, chopped
½ red bell pepper, chopped (optional)
Fresh salmon fillet, about 2 pounds
4 medium garlic cloves
4 rounds of sliced fresh ginger root
2 tablespoons tamari or soy sauce
2 teaspoons toasted sesame oil
2 teaspoons maple syrup (tip: measure the sesame oil first and the syrup won't stick to the spoon)
3 tablespoons lemon juice
2 slices of lemon, seeds removed
2 teaspoons rosemary leaves
1 teaspoon dill weed (dry or fresh)
2 tablespoons chopped fresh basil (or 2 teaspoons dried) (tip: Thai basil is even better, if you can find it.)
½ serrano pepper (optional)
⅛ teaspoon ground nutmeg (optional)

. . . .

1. Set the top rack of the oven to about 6 inches below the broiler flame or coil. Preheat the oven to 375°F.

2. Rinse the kale. On a cutting board, use a sharp knife to cut the leaves across the stems into strips about ⅛ inch wide. You can stack and cut about 6 leaves at a time.

3. Combine the kale and the chopped leek (or onion) and the chopped red bell pepper, if using, in a 9 by 13-inch baking tray. Mix lightly by hand and spread evenly along the bottom of the dish. Sprinkle in ¼ cup of water. This will be a "foundation" for the fish. Set aside.

4. Rinse the fish and pat dry with a paper towel. Place skin-down on a clean cutting board (you may want to put waxed paper on the board first to keep it clean). Using a sharp knife, make diagonal cuts into the fish, about 1 inch apart and to a depth of about half the thickness of the flesh. Turn the board 90 degrees and make cuts in the other direction so that there is a diamond pattern of cuts in the fish flesh. Center the fish on top of the greens in the tray (for black cod, leave some space between the two fillets). Set aside.

5. Prepare a marinade: Put all the remaining ingredients into a blender or (if you are using an immersion blender) into a 2-cup measuring pitcher or steep-sided bowl. Add ¼ cup of water. Blend the ingredients to create a smooth and consistent sauce. You may need to add small amounts of water (1 tablespoon at a time) until the marinade is the consistency of creamy salad dressing.

6. Spread or pour the marinade evenly over the fish. Gently massage it into the slits that were cut into the fish.

7. Put the prepared dish in the preheated oven. Bake until the visible flesh is no longer translucent (20 to 25 minutes, depending on thickness of the fillet). Leave the dish in the oven for the next step.

8. Switch the oven to broil. Broil the dish until there are light brown to coffee-brown highlights on top (5 to 7 minutes). Don't let it burn!

9. Remove the dish from the oven. Let it rest for 3 minutes, then serve hot.

NOTES/TIPS: The optional chopped red bell pepper adds a festive green and red color flair to the kale and leek mixture.

While more expensive, we recommend getting high-quality salmon—wild (not farmed) and with a high fat content, such as Pacific King (Chinook) or Coho. There is controversy about the taste and nutritional balance of farmed fish, including all so-called Atlantic salmon.

BLACK COD VARIANT (LOWER COST): A less costly but equally tasty option is to substitute salmon with 2 pounds (2 fillets) of fresh black cod (also known as sablefish). For this, the first baking time should be reduced to 15 minutes.

GLUTEN-FREE • NUT-FREE • VEGETARIAN • DAIRY-FREE OPTION • VEGAN OPTION

MASHED CAULI-TATOES

Serves 6 as a side dish • Active prep time: 10 minutes • Total time: 30 minutes

Typo? Nope! This tasty side dish is a higher-fiber and lower-blood-sugar impact option for traditional mashed potatoes. It is great for meals that have sauce or

gravy that begs for a "carrier" but for which you don't want to board the blood-sugar roller coaster.

. . . .

4 medium potatoes (I recommend Yukon Gold), cut into 1-inch chunks
½ head of cauliflower, cut into 1-inch chunks
2 garlic cloves, cut in half (optional)

1 teaspoon rosemary leaves (optional)
½ teaspoon salt
¼ cup milk or milk substitute
2 tablespoons butter or olive oil

. . . .

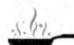

1. Put the potatoes, cauliflower, and garlic and rosemary, if using, into a 2-quart saucepan. Add water to barely cover. Place over high heat.
2. Bring the pot to a boil, then lower the heat and cook the vegetables until tender, 12 to 15 minutes.
3. Drain the water from the pot, using a colander if needed.
4. Into the pot of hot vegetables, add the salt, milk, and butter or oil.
5. Use a potato masher or large spoon to mash and blend all the ingredients in the pot to a creamy consistency.
6. Transfer to a serving dish and serve hot.

GLUTEN-FREE · VEGAN

OVEN-ROASTED VEGETABLE SNACKS

Serves 4 as a snack or side dish • Active prep time: 10 minutes • Total time: 30 minutes

We started roasting vegetables to make simple, low-calorie side dishes or snack options. The prep time is minimal, and the flavors are great. Select your favorite options from the ingredients list to create your version of dozens of potential combinations!

VEGETABLE OPTIONS

PICK YOUR FAVORITES TO GET TO 6 CUPS

Asparagus, in 2-inch lengths

Bell peppers, in ½-inch strips

Broccoli, in about 1-inch chunks

Broccolini, in 2-inch lengths

Brussels sprouts, cut into quarters

Carrots, cut into 2-inch sticks

Cauliflower, in about 1-inch chunks

Fennel bulb, in ½-inch strips

Onion, in ½-inch strips

Yams, sliced into 2-inch "fries"

Zucchini, in ¼-inch-thick rounds

BASIC SEASONING

1 tablespoon olive oil

½ teaspoon salt

2 teaspoons lemon juice or balsamic vinegar

OPTIONAL SEASONING, TO TASTE

½ teaspoon garlic granules

1 teaspoon turmeric powder

¼ teaspoon ground black pepper

½ teaspoon dried oregano

¼ teaspoon ground cayenne pepper

¼ teaspoon ground nutmeg

½ teaspoon dried tarragon

1. Preheat the oven to 400°F.

2. Put your vegetable selections into a large mixing bowl.

3. Add the olive oil, salt, lemon juice or vinegar, and your selection of optional seasonings. Toss with tongs or a large spoon until the veggies are well seasoned and lightly covered with oil.

4. Turn the seasoned vegetables out onto a baking tray lined with parchment paper. Spread evenly in one layer.

5. Roast until the vegetables are tender, about 20 minutes.

6. Remove from the oven and let cool.

7. Enjoy as a snack, appetizer, or side dish.

STORAGE TIP: Once roasted and cooled, the vegetables can be refrigerated in a sealed container. To reduce wilting, fold a paper towel and put it in the container underneath the vegetables.

GLUTEN-FREE • NUT-FREE • VEGAN

QUINOA TABOULI

Serves 6 as a side dish • Active prep time: 30 minutes • Total time: 30 minutes

This is a fresh and fun salad for the spring and summer that has a nice blend of starch and fiber. As with any salad, it is best not to add any salt (or ingredients that contain salt) to the dish until it is ready to serve because the salt will wilt the fresh leaves. If you plan to store the salad and eat it in small servings, salt each serving separately. I enjoy this dish garnished with cherry tomatoes (each cut in half).

I strongly advise using a food processor to prepare this dish, as it otherwise requires a lot of chopping. This recipe is written for food-processor preparation.

2 cups dry quinoa (I prefer red quinoa)
4 mint tea teabags
2 large lemons, rinsed
5 garlic cloves
½ serrano pepper (optional)
1 medium onion, cut into quarters

2 bunches of Italian (flat-leaf) parsley
2 cups fresh mint leaves
4 medium carrots, rinsed
⅓ cup extra-virgin olive oil
½ teaspoon ground black pepper
  (optional)

GARNISH (PER SERVING)

¼ teaspoon Maldon sea salt

6 cherry tomatoes, cut in half

Cook the quinoa at least 3 hours ahead

1. Put 1¾ cups of water into a 2-quart saucepan with a good lid and set to boil over high heat.

2. When the water is at a rolling boil, add the teabags, then the quinoa. Bring back to a full boil, then cover with the lid and lower the heat to simmer. Set a timer for 16 minutes. DO NOT OPEN THE LID during the cooking time.

3. After 16 minutes, turn off the heat but do not open the lid. Set the pot aside to cool for at least 1 hour. After the hour, remove and dispose of the used teabags.

Make the salad

1. Juice the lemons. Set the juice aside. Take one of the empty lemon rinds and cut out 2 strips, each about 1 inch by ½ inch. Save these strips for the next step.

2. Set up the food processor with a sharp chopping blade.

   a) Turn the processor on and drop in the garlic, strips of lemon rind, and serrano pepper. if using. When the food is finely minced, turn off the processor and leave the minced food in it.

   b) Add the onion to the food processor and "pulse chop" until chopped but not pulped. Empty the entire contents of the food processor into a 6-quart mixing bowl.

   c) Now put the parsley and mint leaves into the food processor. "Pulse chop" them until the pieces are fine but not mealy or pulped. Add this to the mixing bowl.

3. Set up the food processor for "coarse grating." Grate the carrots and add them to the mixing bowl.

4. Add the cooked cooled quinoa, reserved lemon juice, olive oil, and black pepper to the bowl. Use a large spoon to stir everything until well mixed.

5. Garnish with the sea salt and tomatoes and serve.

NOTES/TIPS: After cooking the quinoa, if it will be more than 4 hours before you prepare the salad, then either refrigerate the cooled cooked quinoa in a storage container or put the entire saucepan in the fridge. The cooked quinoa can be stored refrigerated for up to 48 hours.

GLUTEN-FREE • NUT-FREE

YATES GONZALEZ FAMILY PAELLA

Serves 8 as a main dish • Active prep time: 45 minutes • Total time: 75 minutes

Paella, a traditional Spanish dish, is as variable and personalized as gumbo or jambalaya or chicken soup. There are a million ways to make it. This is one set

of guidelines for you to make it YOUR way, but almost everything in this recipe is merely a suggestion! Feel free to adjust or tweak things to work for you. Creating the ingredients list was a bit of a challenge since there are many alternatives.

Paella can be made in any size . . . from an individual serving to massive party-size paellas that serve 20 people or more. This recipe is sized for a paella pan 15 inches in diameter with 8 servings.

FOR THE SOFRITO
- 1 large pinch of saffron
- 1 small pinch of sugar (a little less than ⅛ teaspoon)
- 1 pint chicken stock
- ½ cup roasted tomato sauce
- ½ cup port wine or red wine
- 3 bay leaves
- 1 teaspoon Spanish paprika picante
- 1–2 dried hot peppers (optional)

FOR THE PAELLA BASE
- 3 cups paella rice (see note "About paella rice")
- ½ stick (4 tablespoons) of butter or ghee
- 2 tablespoons olive oil
- 6 garlic cloves, chopped fine
- ½ tablespoon chopped rosemary
- 1 large red bell pepper, chopped
- 1 poblano chili, chopped
- 1 serrano chili, chopped (optional)
- 1 large sweet onion, chopped
- 1 large leek, chopped
- 1 large bunch of lacinato ("dino") kale
- 3 slices of lemon, seeds removed
- Garnish: 1 bunch parsley, chopped

FOR THE PAELLA PROTEIN
SELECT ANY 3 PROTEINS (SEE NOTE "ABOUT SELECTING PROTEINS")

- 10 ounces boneless skinless chicken thighs (3 small or 2 large), cut into 1-inch chunks
- Optional addition: 2 small "chubs" Bilbao chorizo (3 ounces total). Remove casing, cut in half lengthwise, then in thin slices.
- 10–12 ounces swordfish (1 "steak" ½ to ¾ inch thick and the size of a tea saucer), cut into cubes. Swordfish is best but halibut, cod, mahi-mahi, or many others work fine.
- 10–12 ounces medium shrimp, shelled and deveined
- 8–10 mussels or clams
- 8–10 ounces calamari, cleaned

ABOUT PAELLA RICE: Paella rice is different from other types of rice, and there are many kinds. We suggest you use a paella rice that recommends a 2:1 liquid-to-rice ratio. Using other types of rice (jasmine, Carolina, basmati, brown, short grain, long grain) will yield unpredictable results.

ABOUT SELECTING PROTEINS: Many combinations of seafood or meats can be used in a paella. Going for more than three or four at once makes the dish chaotic and difficult to fit in the pan. Allergies must be accounted for in selecting proteins.

The quantities in this recipe assume you are using three proteins (plus the optional chorizo addition). Adjust amounts if selecting more or fewer than three. Putting in too much will overflow the pan!

Preparation work

Making paella is all about the prep work. If you don't have things prepared and laid out before you turn on a burner, you will be stressed trying to make this come together. Please take time to do all the following:

1. For the sofrito, prepare the saffron. Keep the saffron dry until it is powdered. Put the pinch of saffron into the smallest glass bowl or ramekin you can find. Add the pinch of sugar. Use the back of a spoon to grind the saffron and sugar into a fine powder. Add 1 teaspoon of water to this and set aside carefully (the liquid will stain anything it spills onto). This tincture needs to sit for 20 minutes while you do the rest of the prep work.

2. For the paella, measure out the 3 cups of rice and set aside.

3. Rinse and cut the kale. On a cutting board, use a sharp knife to cut the leaves across the stems into strips about ⅛ inch wide. You can stack and cut about 6 leaves at a time. Set aside.

4. Cut up the remaining vegetables and your three selected proteins as indicated and set them aside. Don't expect to do this "on the fly."

Start the sofrito

1. Put all the sofrito ingredients into a dry 2-quart saucepan, including the saffron

tincture you prepared earlier. Set the pan to boil over medium heat. The target is for this to be just at a boil in about 15 minutes.

Assemble and cook the paella

1. Preheat the oven to 375°F. It will be about 20 minutes until you need the oven.

2. Place the paella pan on the largest burner you can. In some cases, you may want to have it across two burners for more even heat distribution.

3. In the paella pan, melt the butter over high heat. Add the olive oil. When the combined fats are hot, add the chopped garlic, chopped rosemary, and chopped fresh peppers. Sauté for 2 minutes, then add the chopped onions. Sauté for 4 minutes, then add the chopped leeks.

4. Once the vegetables have cooked down, after 4 minutes:
   a) Shake the paella rice into the still-cooking vegetables. Stir until the mixture is even.
   b) If you are using chicken, add it to the mixture now.
   c) If using the optional Bilbao chorizo, add it now.
   d) Add the kale. Stir carefully, as the pan will be pretty full.

5. Cook the mixture in the pan at high heat, stirring frequently, for 2 to 3 minutes (until the rice starts to lightly toast and the kale is wilted).

6. By now the sofrito soup should be at a low boil. Carefully pour it into the paella pan. It will sizzle and steam as it combines with the sauté. Stir the pan ONCE to get an even distribution, then let it settle. Insert the lemon slices. DO NOT STIR THIS ANYMORE!

7. Turn the paella pan heat to medium. It should continue to boil/bubble but not burn on the bottom. Let it cook without stirring it until the liquid is below the level of the rice but the rice is still wet (10 to 15 minutes).

8. Now comes the tricky part: Use a tablespoon to make small pockets in the rice mixture and drop your seafood elements (chunks or pieces or shells) into these pockets one at a time. Do this quickly but steadily. If you're feeling ambitious, artfully arrange the shellfish.

9. When you have placed all the protein in the paella dish, turn off the stovetop and move the whole pan to the top shelf of the hot oven (375°F).

Bake for 12 to 15 minutes, or until the seafood elements are no longer translucent.

10. Remove from the oven and garnish with a good layer of the chopped parsley on top of the dish.

11. Let it rest for 5 minutes. Set on the table to serve. Enjoy!

ABOUT THE SPICE LEVEL: Our family prefers food to be strongly spiced. This recipe as written turns out to be about a "medium" spice level at a typical Indian or Thai restaurant. Dial down the spicy stuff if you prefer.

This recipe is higher in fiber than many traditional recipes, which works well for us. You may wish to modify the recipe to omit some of the green things.

ONE-POT MEAL · DAIRY-FREE · GLUTEN-FREE · NUT-FREE

NO-FUSS CHICKEN AND LENTILS

Serves 4 as a main dish • Active prep time: 30 minutes • Total time: 90 minutes

(Adapted from *The New York Times*) This one-pot chicken and lentil recipe takes a well-spiced blend of pantry staples plus a handful of fresh ingredients and combines them for a single-pot meal that is both comforting and filling.

2 tablespoons olive oil
6 bone-in, skin-on chicken thighs
    (1½ to 2 pounds), patted dry
2 medium carrots, cut into rounds
1 onion, sliced thin
2 tablespoons tomato paste
1 tablespoon ground cumin
1 teaspoon ground turmeric

2 garlic cloves, minced
1 cup green lentils, rinsed
1 pint chicken stock
Salt and pepper
1 lemon, halved
2 tablespoons chopped cilantro or
    parsley leaves

1. Heat the oil in a large Dutch oven or pot over medium-high heat until shimmering.

2. Brown the chicken, skin side down, in the oil for 7 to 9 minutes. Remove the chicken from the pan and set aside.

3. Add the carrots and onions to the (now chicken-flavored) oil and cook until softened, 3 minutes. Add the tomato paste, cumin, turmeric, and garlic and cook for 2 more minutes.

4. Return the chicken and its juices back to the pot. Add the lentils, 2 cups of water, and the chicken stock.

5. Adjust the heat to bring the liquid to a boil, and season with the salt. Cover with the lid slightly ajar, adjust the heat to a simmer, and cook, stirring occasionally, until the lentils are tender, the chicken is cooked through, and the flavors are blended, 40 to 45 minutes.

6. Stir in half of the lemon juice. Spoon the sauce over the chicken, then taste and season as needed with more lemon juice or salt. Finish with a few grinds of pepper, and sprinkle with the cilantro before serving.

NUT-FREE · GLUTEN-FREE · VEGAN OPTION

CHICKPEAS WITH SPINACH

Serves 3 as a side dish • Active prep time: 10 minutes • Total time: 25 minutes

1 tablespoon olive oil
1 medium onion, chopped
2 garlic cloves, minced
½ teaspoon grated ginger root
1 teaspoon ground cumin seeds
1 tablespoon tomato paste
Sea salt
One 15-ounce can chickpeas

(retain ¼ cup of the liquid, called aquafaba)
1 cup chicken or vegetable stock
Smoked paprika, to taste
One 6-ounce bag of spinach
Ground black pepper, to taste

1. Heat the olive oil in a large, heavy saucepan over medium heat and add the onion. Cook, stirring, until tender, about 5 minutes.

2. Add the garlic, ginger, cumin, tomato paste, and ½ teaspoon sea salt. Cook,

stirring, for 1 to 2 minutes, until fragrant and the tomato paste has turned a darker color.

3. Add the chickpeas and ¼ cup of the retained liquid (aquafaba), the stock, and paprika, and bring to a simmer. Cover, reduce the heat, and simmer for 12 minutes.

4. Add the spinach, cover, and cook until the spinach wilts, about 1 minute. Stir the wilted spinach.

5. Add sea salt and pepper to taste and serve.

DAIRY-FREE · GLUTEN-FREE · NUT-FREE

SOOTHING CHICKEN SOUP

Serves 4 as a main dish • Active prep time: 15 minutes • Total time: 45 minutes

This flavorful soup recipe is warming, soothing, and can be used in lots of ways. It can be the base for other meals or a "catchall" where you can add whatever leftovers you have in your refrigerator to avoid wasted food and make a quick meal.

2 tablespoons olive oil
1 large onion, diced
1 cup chopped celery
2 tablespoons chopped fresh ginger
4–8 garlic cloves, roughly chopped
4 cups chicken stock
1 teaspoon sea salt

⅛ teaspoon cayenne pepper
2 bay leaves
1 cup leafy greens (bok choy, spinach, mustard greens, kale, etc.)
1½ pounds chicken thighs
Juice of half a lemon (or to taste)

GARNISH
¼ cup scallions, cilantro, or parsley, chopped

1 pinch of chili flakes
1 teaspoon toasted sesame oil (optional)

1. Gently heat the oil in a 4-quart soup pot over medium heat. Do not let the oil burn. Add the onion, celery, ginger, and garlic and sauté until fragrant, 3

to 4 minutes. Lower the heat to medium-low and continue sautéing until golden, 3 to 4 more minutes.

2. Add the chicken stock, 2 cups of water, the sea salt, cayenne pepper, bay leaves, leafy greens, and chicken to the pot. Bring to a boil. Cover with a lid and lower the heat. Gently simmer for 20 minutes.

3. Test a piece of chicken for doneness by pulling the meat apart with two forks. It should come apart easily and look opaque. If it is done, shred the rest of the chicken by pulling it apart with forks, then return to the pot and simmer gently for 5 more minutes.

4. Add the lemon juice to the soup, taste, and adjust with more lemon juice if preferred. Add more salt if needed, or if it's too salty for your taste, water it down a little. Adding a starch like rice, noodles, or beans will decrease the salty taste, so go easy on the salt until you have the flavor you prefer.

5. Garnish with chili flakes, scallions, cilantro, or parsley. If you choose, add a drizzle of toasted sesame oil on each bowl just before eating. It adds a savory bit of smokiness.

NOTES/TIPS: As always, "test, don't guess." Check your blood sugar if you add a starch like rice, noodles, or beans to this soup so that you know how your body responds to this meal and the food combinations.

If you really want noodles and want to avoid blood sugar spikes, buy or make zucchini "noodles." You can use a spiralizer attachment on a KitchenAid mixer or a similar device to make noodles from fresh zucchini. These zucchini noodles are delicious and avoid the blood sugar impact that might come with using wheat or rice noodles.

DAIRY-FREE · NUT-FREE · GLUTEN-FREE

SIMPLE LEAFY GREENS AND PROTEIN BREAKFAST

Serves 1 • Active prep time: 10 minutes • Total time: 15 minutes

This is a tasty and hearty breakfast that includes leafy greens and no grains.

4 to 6 leaves Swiss chard, chopped (use
   more if desired)
¼ onion, or 2 tablespoons chopped
   scallions
¼ teaspoon granulated garlic

¼ teaspoon ground cumin
4 ounces salmon, precooked or smoked,
   or canned sardines, or precooked
   shrimp
1 tablespoon olive oil

1. Steam together 4 to 6 leaves or more of the chopped chard, chopped onion
   or scallion, granulated garlic, and ground cumin.

2. Stir the precooked salmon (or canned sardines or precooked shrimp) into the
   steamed chard mix.

3. Drizzle the olive oil over the food after you are done with the cooking.

4. Eat up! Yum!

GLUTEN-FREE • VEGAN

CHOCOLATE-AVOCADO PUDDING

Serves 6 as a dessert • Active prep time: 10 minutes • Total time: 40 minutes

This no-added-sugar dessert is delicious and a simple way to feel satisfied after
eating. If you struggle with satiety or portion control, this recipe is a help.

1 avocado
¼ cup semisweet chocolate chips
¼ cup cacao powder (or cocoa powder
   with no added sugar)

2 tablespoons to ¼ cup unsweetened
   almond milk
1 teaspoon vanilla extract

GARNISH (OPTIONAL)
Sliced strawberries, pecans, or sunflower seeds

1. Slice, pit, and peel the avocado. Put into a food processor or blender.

2. Melt the chocolate chips in the microwave in a microwave-safe bowl in 15-second intervals, adding splashes of water as needed to keep the consistency smooth.

3. Add the melted chocolate chips to the food processor along with the cacao powder, 2 tablespoons of the almond milk, and the vanilla extract.

4. Blend the ingredients together until smooth, adding more almond milk as needed.

5. Pour the creamy rich mousse evenly into 6 small dessert cups for you and your friends to enjoy right away, or store in the fridge for a cold but sweet treat later.

6. Garnish as desired by topping with sliced strawberries, pecans, or sunflower seeds.

DAIRY-FREE · GLUTEN-FREE · VEGAN

3-INGREDIENT CHIA-SEED PUDDING

Serves 2 • Active prep time: 5 minutes • Total time: 2 hours

This 3-Ingredient Chia Pudding is quick, easy, and tasty. This recipe uses nut, seed, or oat "milk" (non-dairy beverages that are alternatives to cow's milk), chia seeds, and added fruit, seeds, or nuts of choice. It's a healthy dessert or snack loaded with protein, fiber, and healthy fats.

There is no need for added sugar. If you prefer to sweeten the pudding, you can add toppings like fresh fruit, dried fruit, or chocolate chips (or leave out the toppings; it's your choice).

2 tablespoons chia seeds
½ cup almond milk or non-dairy milk-
like beverage of choice—read the
label to be sure there are no added

sugars or sweeteners in the
beverage
Blueberries or other fruits for topping
Nuts or other seeds for topping

1. Put 1 tablespoon of the chia seeds and ¼ cup of the nondairy beverage into each of two 8-ounce mason jars. Screw on the lids and shake well.

2. Let the mixtures settle for 2 to 3 minutes, then shake again to mix thoroughly. The mixtures should still be very runny, but if mixed well, you won't see any clumps of chia seeds anywhere in the jar.

3. Put the lidded mason jars in the fridge for at least 2 hours or up to 7 days. The chia seeds will absorb all the liquid, firming up the pudding and making it ready to eat.

4. When you're ready to eat it, top with your favorite fruit, nuts, or seeds and enjoy the cold refreshing dessert!

NOTES/TIPS: You will need two clear 8-ounce mason jars with tight-fitting lids. These are often used for canning preserves or jelly. The chia pudding fills up about half the jar, leaving room for toppings like fresh fruit, nuts, or seeds if you'd like to add them.

The ratio is everything! There are different recommendations for chia pudding out there. Our family has found that 2 tablespoons of chia seeds for every ½ cup of non-dairy milk-like beverage works best. Adjust the ratios to find the consistency you like best.

III

Deeper Dives

CHAPTER 9

Blood Sugar Science

How It Works and Why Act Now

CHAPTER MAP

This chapter explains how blood sugar works, the dangers of high blood sugar—even if you "just" have prediabetes—and why it's never too late to fix it and reclaim health.

KEY SECTIONS

- The science of high blood sugar and its devastating effects
- How type 2 diabetes happens: first insulin resistance, then pancreatic insufficiency
- Insulin resistance: Don't hesitate to act
- Prediabetes: Take action NOW

The fluorescent lights flickered as Jack stared up at the ceiling and blinked tears out of his eyes. He'd just looked down and seen the bandages on his foot. Two weeks ago, he walked out of his doctor's office with a decent bill of health. Sure, his blood sugar numbers hadn't come back great, *but they were stable. A few days later he'd gotten a blister on one of his toes.* Okay . . . no big deal, *he'd thought. He'd put a Band-Aid on and forgotten all about it. But it had gotten infected and worsened quickly. And now here he was: two weeks later, in a hospital bed with one less toe.*

Jack's surgeon told him he was lucky. Sometimes people lose their whole foot, or even part of their leg. People with diabetes suffer from blood vessel damage and impaired circulation to the extremities, along with compromised immune system function, meaning they are at greater risk of infections, which can lead to amputations. In fact, they are thirty times more likely to require amputation. That's a big, preventable, increase in relative risk. Jack went on to focus on reducing his stress and commit to meal timing so he could avoid the exaggerated dawn phenomenon that kept his blood sugar from returning to healthy levels when he awakened each day.

I met Jack shortly after this tragic incident. He was in a high-risk position. He'd already suffered from the dangers of high blood sugar. But it's never too late to stop the train of harm and turn it around. Diabetes and high blood sugar usually keep worsening when left unaddressed. I started my work with Jack by asking myself the question: What are his opportunities for healing?

There is always something we can do. The body is resilient. It heals and restores wellness when nourished, sometimes astoundingly quickly.

We made a few key changes to his eating patterns. He made sure to eat dinner at least 4–5 hours before bedtime, he added leafy greens to all meals, and he stopped skipping lunch to avoid overeating at dinnertime.

It's a sad fact: Type 2 and prediabetes have become so common that our culture is blasé about the dangers. We've normalized them. *Oh, you've got type 2? Me too!* We've stopped thinking of them as life-threatening conditions. But the risks are huge. It's very serious. And the damage of high blood sugar is always happening, even if your case isn't severe.

In this chapter, I describe how blood sugar works and why high blood sugar is so devastating, but also the good news: You're never doomed. Even if you're at high risk like Jack, you can reverse the trajectory. You can always support your vulnerable areas. Any damage to your metabolic machinery is also an opportunity for healing and reversal. It's an opportunity to get out of blood sugar danger zones and into better health, energy, and freedom.

THE SCIENCE OF HIGH BLOOD SUGAR AND ITS DEVASTATING EFFECTS

Sugar naturally rises and falls in the blood.

But for people with type 2 and prediabetes, blood sugar levels remain higher, longer.

Sugar is sticky. Think of the difference between water and syrup, or how hard it is to clean up spilled juice compared to water. Sugar sticks to proteins and fats in a process called *glycation*.

Glycation gums up the blood. It gets thick and sticky, so it does not move as freely. A cardiologist might refer to this as impaired perfusion, or compromised blood flow. You need your blood to flow so it can deliver nutrients and pick up the natural waste products. If this flow is disrupted, you become more vulnerable to issues related to glycation.

Glycation creates a group of toxic by-products called AGEs (advanced glycation end products). AGEs are like little gummy pickaxes. In the blood, they can pile up, further reducing blood flow and damaging blood vessels. As they circulate around the body, they ravage every part of you: every kind of tissue, every organ. No part of the body is safe from AGEs. AGEs have been associated with premature aging, heart disease, kidney failure, declining memory, eye disease, polycystic ovary syndrome (PCOS), impaired wound healing, cardio-vascular complications, impaired bone health, periodontitis, erectile dysfunction, peripheral neuropathy, peripheral artery disease, obstructive sleep apnea, cancer, schizophrenia, dementia, and Alzheimer's (plus others). AGEs can even kill cells that cannot be replaced, causing permanent damage. A meta-analysis demonstrated increased risk of death from all causes with higher circulating AGEs.

The damage from high blood sugar begins as early as blood sugar levels start to rise. Much of it is silent and invisible. It can build up for years before you notice symptoms, or your doctor decides to intervene. The most common places it affects are the kidneys, eyes, nervous system, and cardiovascular system. Each person's vulnerabilities depend on their genetics and what's happened in their life. We are not equally vulnerable to the same things. Glycation, like other system-wide issues such as inflammation, makes a beeline for the weakest link.

Kidney damage (nephropathy)

Approximately 1 in 3 adults with diabetes, both type 1 and type 2, has kidney disease. Kidneys are made of small units called nephrons. Nephrons filter the blood, remove waste from the body, and control fluid balance. In diabetes, nephrons thicken and become scarred over time, resulting in leakage and an impaired ability to filter the blood. Diabetes also causes the bladder to function at lower capacity, resulting in difficulty emptying the bladder and a backlog of waste that the kidneys struggle to eliminate.

Nephropathy can lead to kidney failure, meaning needing dialysis for life or a kidney transplant. More than 200,000 people with end-stage kidney failure due to diabetes are on dialysis or have had a kidney transplant. Diabetes is the most common cause of end-stage kidney failure. Kidney failure increases the likelihood of death from other causes. Kidney damage is also one of the strongest predictors of death or other adverse outcomes when people experiencing heart failure are admitted or rushed to the hospital.

Vision damage

Glycation reduces blood flow to the eyes, causing vision loss, and when AGEs accumulate in the eye, they lead to vision impairment, cataracts, and eventually blindness. Five percent of people with diabetes suffer severe vision loss. Seventy-eight percent of people with type 2 are expected to develop at least some retinal damage after having diabetes for fifteen years. The structural changes in the eye can be irreversible.

Nerve cell death (neuropathy) and amputation

Glycation kills nerve cells. This damage can cause pain, numbness, tingling, swelling, or muscle weakness in different parts of the body, usually beginning in the hands or feet and worsening over time.

Peripheral neuropathy is the death of nerve cells in the periphery: in the hands and feet. When nerve cells die in conjunction with the gummed-up blood flow and decreased oxygen, cells become hypoxic from the lack of oxygen, and ulcers form. Ulcers can cause severe damage to tissue and bone or can become infected from the effects diabetes has on the immune system. This is why Jack's toe needed to be amputated.

Every year, 154,000 Americans with diabetes undergo amputation.

Nerve cells are also responsible for coordinating internal functions such as digestion, so diabetic neuropathy causes symptoms such as urinary incontinence, diarrhea, and constipation.

Heart and blood vessel damage

AGEs negatively affect cardiovascular health in several ways, including by contributing to arterial stiffening, a key risk factor for heart disease. They also contribute to cardiac dysfunction, where the lower heart chambers don't relax as they should, ultimately leading to heart failure.

This kind of dysfunction has been directly linked to elevated A1C levels and AGEs. It is present in 50 to 60 percent of type 2 diabetes patients.

Forty percent of people with diabetes experience heart failure. Men with diabetes are two times more likely to experience heart failure than men without it; women are five times more likely.

The longer you have diabetes, the more likely you are to develop heart disease. The presence of diabetes has been shown to increase the risk of death or hospitalization due to heart failure by 200 percent for insulin users and 50 percent for non-insulin treated patients.

Brain, memory, and mood damage

High blood sugar impacts the brain. AGEs are associated with increased risk of developing dementia and Alzheimer's; researchers are currently exploring the link between type 2 and Alzheimer's; sometimes Alzheimer's is called type 3 diabetes.

People with diabetes are two to three times more likely to have depression. Insulin resistance increases the risk of depression by 200 percent. Recent studies have suggested that the presence of AGEs predicts/increases the risk of mental health disorders, especially schizophrenia and depression. AGEs appear to predict schizophrenia and psychosis in adolescents, and higher AGE levels appear to correlate with depressive symptoms.

Immune and reproductive health damage

There are other damaging and dangerous effects of type 2 and prediabetes. The associated inflammation dysregulates the immune system. It also impairs hormone function. For example, excess insulin causes female reproductive organs to overproduce testosterone, leading to polycystic ovary syndrome (PCOS), the most common cause of infertility in the United States. High insulin in concordance with hypertension and other factors results in higher rates of erectile dysfunction, delayed ejaculation, and low sperm count in men.

WHAT IS DIABETES?

Why do blood sugar levels remain higher, longer for people with prediabetes and type 2?

Sugar is a natural element of the blood and body chemistry. It's so important that if you don't consume it, the body makes its own.

But too much sugar is toxic. If you exceed 600 mg/dl of sugar in your blood, you can enter a diabetic coma and die. The body has metabolic machinery in place that tightly regulates sugar levels. This metabolic machinery includes the liver, the pancreas, muscles, fat tissue, and even the immune system, the gut, and the brain.

The key organ in this machinery is the pancreas. When the pancreas detects sugar in the blood, it produces a hormone called insulin. Hormones are messenger molecules. Insulin's job is to tell muscle, fat, and liver cells that they need to open up and let sugar in.

Diabetes is when this process stops working effectively. It's when your body can't get sugar into storage. Blood sugar stays in the blood higher and longer than is good for you. It undergoes the glycation process and gums up the blood and produces those toxic AGEs.

Type 1 diabetes is a result of autoimmune damage to the pancreas. The beta cells in the pancreas that produce insulin get permanently damaged. They can't make the insulin needed to move blood sugar into storage. Type 1 diabetics must inject insulin to make up for this. They must monitor blood sugar and inject the right amount of insulin to keep levels in a healthy range. If they don't, they can die.

Type 2 diabetes is different from type 1 because it develops progressively over time. It can take many years, even decades, to reach the tipping point of serious need where health professionals finally, sometimes too late, consider intervention necessary. Like type 1, the beta cells in the pancreas that produce insulin are damaged, and sometimes die. But unlike type 1, the damage isn't total and permanent. Healthy functioning can be preserved and possibly restored.

If you implement the steps and heal the damage to the metabolic machinery, you restore some if not all the original functionality of this system.

HOW TYPE 2 DIABETES HAPPENS: FIRST INSULIN RESISTANCE, THEN PANCREATIC INSUFFICIENCY

In simplified and generalized terms, people usually develop type 2 diabetes in a two-step process.

First is the development of insulin resistance. Insulin resistance is when the cells that are supposed to store blood sugar—fat, muscle, and especially liver cells—lose their capacity to properly respond to insulin's signal that it's time to store it. They have sites on their surfaces intended to receive this signal. These sites can become damaged by things like inflammation, which makes them resistant to insulin's signal.

When cells start to become insulin resistant, the pancreas produces more insulin. More insulin is the only way to get the cells to be able to hear the signal. If sugar levels continue to rise unchecked, you could become comatose and die. The pancreas goes into hyperdrive. It's like a fire station trying to put out a raging fire. It just keeps sending more fire trucks.

Often, and especially early in the progression of type 2 and prediabetes, the pancreas makes a lot of insulin and succeeds at forcing blood sugar into storage. But it takes more insulin than is healthy. Sometimes the pancreas keeps up with the increased demand to send all these fire trucks. It keeps going on hyperdrive for as long as it needs, keeping blood sugar levels within a relatively healthy range.

But usually, it can't keep up. It has performed its job on hyperdrive while under assault from inflammation and other sources of damage. The demand on it has continued to increase while accruing damage on several fronts. It begins to lag behind.

This is the second phase of developing type 2 diabetes: pancreatic insufficiency—aka exhaustion. The pancreas stops being able to keep up. The body finally enters a diabetic state, where it just can't get as much blood sugar out of the blood as it needs to. Blood sugar levels stay too high too long. Complications like blood vessel damage, heart damage, brain damage, kidney damage, and retina damage have been underway all along, and now the risks are significant.

CRASHING OR RUNAWAY HIGHS

Early on in the progression from insulin resistance to prediabetes and type 2, blood sugar crashes are common. They happen when the pancreas floods the blood with as much insulin as possible. It's been doing this dance for a while and knows that it needs to overproduce insulin to wrestle that blood sugar into storage. It overshoots, so you crash. It's a blood-sugar roller coaster, rocketing up and slamming you down the other side.

When you crash, you can be dizzy, lightheaded, exhausted, shaky, in a low mood with low energy, irritable, "hangry," anxious, and have a big appetite even though you're not genuinely hungry. You're exhausted even though you consciously haven't physically done anything. Your organs have done a lot. Sometimes people rocket up to a blood sugar level of about 250 mg/dl, then plummet back down to around 70. This can leave you feeling unwell and out of sorts.

Later in the progression of developing diabetes, crashes can become less common because the pancreas starts lagging behind. When this happens, blood sugar levels stay up in dangerous ranges for even longer than before. You could rocket up by 100 points and stay there or come down only slowly. This is one reason it is so important on the Yates Protocol to eat proper meals, to avoid snacking, to exercise, and to keep moving throughout the day. When you do these practices, you help bring your numbers down. Over time, this lightens some of the burden on the metabolic machinery. It heals and regains its original functionality.

THE PROGRESSION: INSULIN RESISTANCE TO PREDIABETES TO TYPE 2 DIABETES

Insulin resistance, prediabetes, and type 2 typically worsen. They rarely improve on their own or just stay in a steady state. Compromised vasculature, AGEs, oxidative stress, mitochondria dysfunction, inflammation: All these things contribute to one another. Once you start developing them, they put you on a trajectory that fuels itself. It is a path of more and more damage, into poorer health and increased risk.

Blood sugar levels typically increase *slowly* at the beginning but then pick up speed. You can spend years in insulin resistance or prediabetes with a relatively stable A1C, then all of a sudden it's *up up up*. It's like driving a car with one faulty part: You can keep driving with it, but as it malfunctions, it makes all the other parts around it start to malfunction, too. You drove on it for years and it was okay, but all of a sudden you have not one or two but ten faulty parts on your hands.

INSULIN RESISTANCE: DON'T HESITATE TO ACT

Insulin resistance can precede the clinical diagnosis of type 2 diabetes by up to fifteen years. Typically, changes in blood sugar, insulin sensitivity, and insulin secretion are evident three to six years before a diabetes diagnosis.

The earlier you stop this train, the better off you are. Don't wait until you have prediabetes. How do you know if you are insulin resistant? You may put on weight easily. You may experience blood sugar crashes. If you have a significant body fat percentage, especially visceral fat in and around the abdominal organs, or you live a sedentary life, there's a decent chance you're somewhat insulin resistant. Genes play a major role in how easily you might develop insulin resistance, as well as prediabetes and type 2. If you have an autoimmune condition, joint pain, gut issues, thyroid disease, or chronic fatigue, these all often co-occur with some insulin resistance. If you have a family history, there's an increased chance.

There's a test to help you and your health-care providers get clarity on insulin resistance: fasting insulin. Fasting insulin is a test of your insulin levels after an 8- to 12-hour fast. It's an excellent test and should be a routine part of health checkups.

PREDIABETES: TAKE ACTION NOW

Currently, 1 in 3 American adults—that's 84 million—have prediabetes.

If you are one of them, *now* is the time to act. You have already been developing insulin resistance and damaged metabolic machinery likely for many years. Do not hesitate.

Most people with prediabetes develop type 2 within five years. Without intervention, 5 to 10 percent of people with prediabetes tip over into diabetic every year.

In conventional medicine, practitioners often wait until patients have full-blown type 2 before starting any kind of treatment. Almost all my type 2 patients have stories to tell about how they sat in prediabetes limbo with their doctors for years, doing nothing about it.

Reputable medical institutions state that "Type 2 diabetes is a wake-up call to focus on diet and exercise to try to control our blood sugar and prevent problems."

But this damage is *already happening in prediabetes*. *Prediabetes* is already the *second* wake-up call. Insulin resistance was the first.

Some people with type 2 already have kidney damage when first diagnosed. Prediabetes increases the risk of heart disease and stroke. Damage has already been done. An A1C of 6.5 percent is where many begin to experience symptoms: things like increased thirst, frequent urination, increased hunger, fatigue, blurred vision, numbness or tingling in hands and feet, frequent infections, and slow-healing sores. What causes these symptoms? Damage from AGEs! To be diagnosed as type 2 diabetic means that you have *already been accruing damage from high blood sugar* for years.

The rationale doctors use for waiting to take action until you officially tip over from prediabetic to type 2 is because that is when drugs become "needed." It's when you must intervene because your pancreas can't keep up. If you don't do something dramatic, your blood sugar numbers could put you in the kind of danger that everyone recognizes as an urgent situation. It's when your life becomes at stake: Intervention becomes a matter of life or death.

But why wait to get to this stage?

You can make changes to your diet and lifestyle starting right now that prevent this from happening.

PRO TIP: HEED THE PREDIABETES WAKE-UP CALL

Sandra's A1C had been stable in the prediabetic range at 5.8 percent for years. Her doctor told her to just continue to test annually and watch for increases. Then they'd take action. During a stressful season her A1C went up to 6.6 percent: That's technically type 2 diabetes.

"I wish I could have paid more attention to me," Sandra said. "I thought, **pre**diabetes, 'what's the big deal?' But when you take that little '**pre**' off, ouch."

Today, Sandra is positive and optimistic. She's made changes that have put her type 2 into remission. Her A1C is back in the lower end of the prediabetic range, and I expect it to keep dropping into full reversal.

When I asked if she could go back and tell her prediabetic self anything, Sandra said she'd pay more attention to what her body was telling her.

"This is your wake-up call," she said.

REVERSE THE TRAJECTORY

You aren't doomed! It's all reversible. The process of reversing type 2 and prediabetes is not an overnight switch, but it happens bit by bit. Sometimes, depending on your situation and the changes you make, you can see a difference right away. This is especially likely if you've been eating meals that spike blood sugar and then transition to the nourishing food groups of the Yates Protocol. Once you switch, you will see at least some swift improvement in your post-meal blood sugar numbers. Then it's a matter of staying committed to the process.

In this chapter you learned:

- Excess blood sugar makes the blood sticky, which gums up blood flow and prevents the blood from being able to deliver nutrients and remove waste products. It also creates highly destructive advanced glycation end products (AGEs).

- Each person has different vulnerabilities. High blood sugar affects vulnerable areas first. The most common vulnerable areas are the heart, kidneys, brain, eyes, and nerves.

- High blood sugar can and usually does damage the body for years before effects become severe enough to notice or to get the attention of health-care professionals.

- Type 2 diabetes usually develops in two steps. First is the development of insulin resistance; second is the pancreas lagging behind the increased demand for more and more insulin.

- Prediabetes and insulin resistance are both clear warning signs and signals to act now.

- It's never too late to act. Identify opportunities for healing and seize them.

CHAPTER 10

Causes & Reversal Science

Many Diverse Phenomena Cause the Metabolic Damage Driving Type 2 and Prediabetes. Here's How the Yates Protocol Restores Health

CHAPTER MAP

This chapter explains twelve sources of damage to metabolic machinery that drive the development of type 2 and prediabetes. It concludes in explaining why the Yates Protocol works.

KEY SECTIONS

- Damage, damage everywhere
- It's not your fault
- Why the five steps work
- Choosing what to focus on

Corey looked down and shook his head. "I just don't get it," he said. Many people are shocked and confused when they receive a type 2 or prediabetes diagnosis. Some show signs of weary acceptance as if they were expecting the worst. They'd been trying their hardest to be well. Corey was one of them.

Corey grabbed his laptop, with me on the telehealth app, stood up, and walked into his kitchen. He set the laptop on the counter.

Corey walked to his fridge and cupboards, pulling each open one by one. Thunk, thunk, thunk *they went as their doors gently bumped one another. If even half of his diet was what he kept in here, he was eating great! The fridge was overflowing with fresh vegetables, eggs and meat, and some fruit. The cupboards housed extra-virgin, cold-pressed oils. He had towers of cans of sustainably sourced, wild-caught fish, and glass containers full of organic dry beans and other legumes. I was impressed.*

He shrugged, turned to look me in the eyes, and asked, "What can I do better?"

I invited him to sit down. Then I explained: Sometimes it's not about what you eat.

Corey's prediabetes appeared to be caused by a confluence of a series of unfortunate events. He had just gone through a very stressful divorce. Amidst that stress, he contracted Lyme disease, which triggered latent Epstein–Barr virus. (Sometimes viruses shock the immune system into creating a storm of inflammation that damages the metabolic machinery.) On top of that, inspectors found mold in the home where he was living.

Corey used to have six-pack abs. Now he was prediabetic over the course of just one year. It had nothing to do with how well he ate. His good diet surely helped support his body through the challenges he endured. If he hadn't been eating so well, it would all likely have been worse. But these sources of damage were enough to make the difference.

The science is clear: Reversing type 2 and prediabetes is possible. But how? *Eat less, exercise more* isn't working. *Why not?*

First, we must acknowledge that our understanding of the science is always evolving. I am providing the best knowledge I can, based on my clinical experience and engagement with the scientific literature. *My guidance on this will evolve,* as it's supposed to. This is a defining feature of good science.

Second, we must investigate the root causes. Understand the cause of a problem, then you can do something about it. It's that simple. Type 2 and prediabetes are complex phenomena driven by a variety of causes, but the basic premise remains simple: Understand the damage, then address it.

Many people today presume that type 2 comes from overeating and/or simple laziness, but the truth is you can eat and exercise well and still end up with type 2. The truth is every person's experience of blood sugar is unique. The truth is type 2 and prediabetes are complicated.

When you get curious and explore the individual experiences of individual people, it becomes impossible to paint them with the same brush. You meet people like Corey who struggled with stress and immune system dysregulation, Sonia who rarely got a full night's rest, and Len who spent thirty-one years in *go* mode serving his country. You start to see so many potential causes. You go from one to now dozens or even hundreds of ways to end up in blood sugar danger. These ways are generalizable into different categories, but there is so much variability across individual experiences.

The one common thread is *damage.* All the various causes of type 2 and prediabetes are sources of damage to the metabolic machinery that regulates blood sugar. The Yates Protocol is designed to heal this damage. You implement the five steps. You replenish nutrients, reduce systemic inflammation, and heal the body from mitochondrial dysfunction and oxidative stress. You successfully reverse the damage.

DAMAGE, DAMAGE EVERYWHERE

Type 2 and prediabetes are diseases caused by damage. Major types of damage include, though are not limited to, chronic, systemic inflammation, oxidative stress, and mitochondria dysfunction. Each of these is widespread throughout the body and inflicts damage everywhere, including but not limited to the metabolic machinery.

Inflammation is an important body process. To inflame is to heal. Think of when you get a cut, and it bleeds and swells. The body detects an injury and sends inflammatory molecules to take care of it. This works great for acute injuries. But what happens when the wound is ongoing? Systemic or chronic inflammation is when your body detects a fire it needs to put out but can't.

Chronic (aka systemic) inflammation causes type 2 and prediabetes through two major pathways.

First, it causes insulin resistance. Cells that are supposed to store blood sugar in the liver and muscles (and fat) have receptor sites on their surfaces meant to receive the message from insulin that it's time to let blood sugar in. But when there is an excess of inflammatory markers in the blood, they damage the receptor sites and/or surrounding areas, impairing function. Chronic inflammation makes the cells *resistant* to insulin's message. Pro-inflammatory molecules associated with chronic hyperinflammation, such as inflammatory cytokines, macrophages, C-reactive protein (CRP), high sensitivity C-reactive protein (hs-CRP), and TNF-alpha have been linked to the development of insulin resistance, prediabetes, and type 2.

Second, inflammation damages the beta cells in the pancreas that produce insulin, reducing their capacity to meet the increasing demand for insulin due to insulin resistance. Apoptosis is a natural process in the body where cells die on purpose; the point is to get rid of unneeded or abnormal cells. Certain inflammatory markers (such as interleukin-6 and TNF-alpha) stimulate beta cell apoptosis to dangerous levels. This reduces the capacity of the pancreas to produce insulin, leading to runaway blood-sugar levels and rapidly climbing A1C.

Oxidative stress, like inflammation, causes type 2 diabetes through the two pathways of causing insulin resistance and harming the beta cells that produce insulin. It contributes to insulin resistance by damaging numerous proteins, including ones near the sugar transport channel on cell membranes. And it directly damages beta cells, as they have little natural antioxidant defense.

Oxidative stress is the result of an imbalance between pro-oxidant and antioxidant activity in the body. Pro-oxidant processes are a natural by-product of energy production. They're a necessary evil the body is always working to balance out with antioxidants. This is why eating high-antioxidant vegetables and fruits is so health-promoting. But a diet high in antioxidants can do only so much. When pro-oxidant molecules called reactive oxygen species (ROS) begin to build up, they dominate the antioxidants and cause oxidative stress.

Mitochondrial dysfunction plays a role in type 2 and prediabetes because mitochondria are the powerhouses of cells. They produce the energy cells need to perform their jobs. When mitochondria malfunction, cells, including those involved in producing insulin and managing insulin levels, begin to fail to do their jobs.

Mitochondria moderate the balance between pro-oxidant and antioxidant processes in the body. When mitochondria begin to malfunction, oxidative stress grows. As oxidative stress grows, mitochondria weaken further. It can be a vicious cycle.

And it can worsen other domains of health, because when mitochondria weaken, mental and physical energy both suffer. This makes it more difficult to make healthy choices.

The struggle is quite real.

The various kinds of damage to metabolic machinery are self-reinforcing. Chronic inflammation spurs more oxidative stress and mitochondria malfunction; oxidative stress and mitochondria malfunction spur more chronic inflammation. They can all worsen gut health, bacteria balance in the gut's microbiome, nervous system health, nutrient status, blood flow, the ability to have a healthy stress response, the ability to rest long and deep, metabolic rate, hormone health, and literally everything else.

Sometimes the seed is planted in childhood, and then it takes decades to show. If you've been put on such a bad course, you can eat exactly the same as someone else without diabetes or prediabetes, but you'll get dragged onto a blood-sugar roller coaster ride while they sail along, perfectly fine. It can be so frustrating and confusing. Meanwhile, you're blamed and shamed for something happening to you that absolutely was never your fault to begin with.

Fortunately, even while many remain stuck in the shaming and blaming *eat less, exercise more* model of type 2 and prediabetes, there are plenty of researchers getting to the bottom of the real and diverse causes of damage to the metabolic machinery. Here is a brief overview of twelve major causes of damage (that are presently known).

Genetics

Studies of twins, studies of families, and studies of various racial and ethnic groups across comparable environments suggest that whether you end up with type 2 is highly influenced by the set of genetic predispositions you get at birth. Estimates of heritability range from 25 percent to 80 percent.

Genes do not *predetermine* you. If you've got a lot of type 2 or prediabetes in your family, you're not doomed to get them. Genes influence vulnerability. They create predispositions that can be triggered depending on what happens in your life. There are thousands of different alleles (versions of genes) that can be flipped from off to on by your diet, lifestyle, or environment and increase chances of developing type 2.

Significant recent generational events such as famine, war, displacement, or other major trauma can create *epigenetic* effects, which can predispose you to flip genes to on mode in a way you wouldn't have otherwise.

Then, during your own life the events that can flip them on are nearly too numerous to name, but do include the nutritional status of the womb you began taking shape in, how you were born, if you were breastfed, and what foods and bacteria you were exposed to in these early years. Then how you were nourished throughout your life, how much stress you experienced, how well you've slept, what kinds of activities you've participated in, any medications you've been on, the amount of environmental toxins you may have been exposed to, and so much more have all played a role.

Your experience of type 2 diabetes or prediabetes? Your insulin resistance? Your blood sugar dysregulation? Your hypoglycemia?

All your vulnerabilities? They're not your fault!

Yet, this is also not cause to despair. You can have had alleles flipped to the on position. You can have had significant chronic inflammation, oxidative stress, and decreased function of your insulin signaling and production pathways. *But this damage can be healed.* The genetic switches can be flipped back to off. You will remain vulnerable to their being flipped back to on again, but with intention and healthy habits, you can take control.

The nutrient-poor, inflammatory, hypercaloric, addictive, highly refined, ultra-processed Standard American Diet

There is one way of eating that has conclusively demonstrated itself to be the worst diet for all health outcomes, including type 2 and prediabetes, with the most significant rates of devastation and death we have ever witnessed:

The Standard American Diet.

The Standard American Diet, commonly referred to as the SAD diet, is by far the worst diet on record in human history.

The SAD is characterized by being *ultra-processed*. Minimally processed foods are mostly fresh: vegetables, fruits, and meats. Processed foods are one step above that: e.g., canned beans or fish or yogurt. Ultra-processed foods are a step beyond that and are industrially cooked, designed to be addictive, and synthesized with flavor enhancers, colors, and other additives. They are typically highly caloric, inflammatory, and low in nutrients. They include soda, ice cream, sweets, snacks, breakfast cereals, pizzas, prepared meals, instant noodles, and fast food. Some are worse than others, but they are all full of risk and potential danger.

A recent study cataloging 50,000 food items available in the US food supply suggests that 73 percent of them are ultra-processed. Ultra-processed food is 52 percent cheaper than less processed alternatives, making it a more attractive option for many with lower income. These products are also much more prominent in certain areas of the country and neighborhoods: typically, the poorer ones. In some parts of the US and the world, ultra-processed food is almost all you can find.

Despite the explosion of wellness and diet culture in recent decades, ultra-processed food consumption has risen and continues to rise. A recent analysis of the CDC's National Health and Nutrition Examination Survey (NHANES), which included survey results from 41,000 adults, showed that ultra-processed food consumption grew from 53.5 percent in 2001 to 57 percent in 2018. This was true of people across all demographic groups regardless of income. The one exception was Hispanic adults, who ate significantly less processed foods and more whole foods over this time period.

Adults sixty and over demonstrated the sharpest increase in processed food consumption: In 2001 they ate the least processed and most whole foods; in 2018 they ate the most processed and least whole foods. This is a worrying trend. It could be argued that our elders are the people least able to afford to eat poor-quality food.

SAD foods are designed to be hyperpalatable—aka, way too tasty for our taste buds to handle. It's a devil's brew made by some of the smartest and highest-paid food scientists on the planet, designed to ensnare you on purpose. The human palate is made for the natural world: vegetables, fruits, and animals of the earth, seasoned with herbs, nothing made in a factory. Food companies want you to get addicted.

Step 1 is hijacking taste buds. SAD foods rocket past taste thresholds on purpose and explode the brain's pleasure centers. The right combinations of sugar, unhealthy fats, salt, and other additives flood reward systems designed for comparatively simple sweets like berries, or savory foods like roasted meat.

Defining addiction is thorny and difficult, but the intent with these foods is clearly to make you constantly crave and eat more.

Step 2 is overriding or tricking your natural ability to feel full. Food companies intentionally design foods so you'll consume the most possible before your body can experience satiation. For example, fast-food hamburger buns are designed to require minimal chewing. This makes you eat faster and therefore consume more of the flavors and chemicals in the hamburger designed to addict you before you can get full. In this unnaturally lubricated *chew and swallow* process, you can end up sluicing down a whole burger in minutes if not seconds, maybe along with supersize fries and soda. Your body has not even had a chance to start feeling full and you've already eaten several hundred calories, maybe a thousand or more.

Plus, these foods have little nutrition. Nutrients are satisfying. You can eat a ton of SAD food, but if you never get the nutrients you need, you'll always feel like you need more. SAD foods are biochemically *rewarding*, not *satisfying*. There is a difference. After a SAD meal, since you haven't gotten the nutrients you need, your cravings will likely return stronger and faster.

It is impossible to eat an appropriate amount on SAD foods. But the purveyors of these foods benefit when you think that it *is* possible—so when you fail to do so, it's *your* fault. They'll keep telling you it's your fault and you'll keep drowning in your own supposed shamefulness, all so you can't see what they're doing to you. They pump trillions of dollars into making SAD foods as addictive as possible while insisting you're a lazy sack of potatoes for getting addicted—that is, *for doing exactly what they want you to do.*

It's true that routinely eating a lot more than you need isn't great for you. Excess calorie consumption causes inflammation and oxidative stress. It overburdens the body's fat- and sugar-burning capacities and forces you to operate too much in "energy storage" mode. You end up with too much insulin floating around in your blood too much of the time, making cells more inclined to become more insulin resistant. Chronic intake of excess calories has been shown to engender insulin resistance independent of body fatness.

But excess calorie intake is just *one* of many dangers of the SAD. Hypothetically, let's say you *do* eat the appropriate number of calories of this food. Will you be well? No. Even if you eat the supposedly healthful variants of it—cereal, granola, low-fat yogurts, "green" smoothies—it's all still processed, and most of it is relatively low in nutrients, high in sugar, and high in pro-inflammatory ingredients.

The SAD is full of unhealthy fats such as deep-fried foods, trans fat, and rancid seed oils that contribute to systemic inflammation, oxidative stress, and tissue damage. Almost every ultra-processed meal, condiment, sauce, or dressing is made with such fats—because they're inexpensive and have long shelf lives.

The SAD has added sugar *everywhere*. It's in *everything,* including many items you might not expect, such as hamburger buns, salad dressing, mayonnaise, and almond milk.

Many SAD foods have high amounts of artificial sweeteners. Foods labeled "sugar free" or "no sugar added" or "zero calories" are typically full of artificial sweeteners. These can disrupt insulin signaling, interfere with appetite regulation, and feed harmful gut bacteria that perforate intestinal walls, contribute to intestinal permeability (aka leaky gut syndrome), and prohibit healthy nutrient absorption.

Even processed foods that make health claims on the label, like Heart Healthy Bran Flakes, Low Fat Mayonnaise, or Olive Oil Hummus usually reveal themselves to be wolves in sheep's clothing once you look at the ingredient list.

Plus, how are these foods prepared, in what kinds of packaging, and exposed to what types of cooking methods and materials? This all matters. The more steps a product has to go through to reach you, the more invisible processing it has likely undergone and the more invisible sources of damage it has likely accrued. For example, the high heat processing required for safely cooking and preserving processed protein and carbohydrates creates the advanced glycation end products (AGEs) that contribute to stress and damage across the body. Cooking and storing in plastic containers can result in high amounts of toxic molecules such as BPA, phthalates, or PFAS ("forever chemicals") in even the "healthiest" or most organic processed products.

Wherever the SAD goes, type 2 diabetes and other syndromes associated with major metabolic damage follow. For example, when Australian Aborigines are displaced and move into urban environments, they replace their traditional diets with typical Western food and develop unusually high rates of type 2. These are people who have typically eaten and exercised extremely well throughout life: high-fiber, high-nutrient foods and high levels of physical activity. It has been suggested that these communities are genetically predisposed to store fat and sugar due to their historical living conditions and patterns of feasting and fasting, and while that *may* have truth to it, I think it's much more likely the stress of displacement alongside transitioning to the SAD that wreaks immediate and absolute havoc on their healthy bodies. The new unnatural environment, poor nutrition, and lifestyle changes are the issue.

Malnourishment

Malnutrition is recognized as a serious cause of type 2 diabetes across the world and accounts for widespread and dangerous complications in regions where access to food is scarce. In such regions, type 2 is often associated with very low body mass indices and low albumin, indicating low protein intake.

The significant malnourishment experienced by people in areas of food scarcity is very real, very dangerous, and must be addressed through improving access to food in these areas.

It is also important to recognize that you do not have to have a low body mass index or body fat percentage to be malnourished or undernourished. Johns Hopkins Medicine defines malnutrition as "the condition that develops when the body is deprived of vitamins, minerals and other nutrients it needs to maintain healthy tissues and organ function." Studies that consider malnutrition under the broader definition show that malnutrition and type 2 diabetes associated with malnutrition can be present among people assessed as overweight and obese. Growing up or sustaining yourself on fast food, French fries, pizza, soda, or even supposed "healthy" meals made with ultra-processed versions of healthy foods can result in significant deficiency in important nutrients, including protein, even while eating high quantities of food.

Visceral body fat

Excess body fat is a significant risk factor for the development of type 2 diabetes. It's true: If you have a high body fat percentage, you are more likely to have type 2. This doesn't mean higher body fat percentages are *the* or even *a* cause of type 2. People with type 2 diabetes can be incredibly lean. And people who carry extra body fat do not always get type 2. So, what's the deal? Body fat does appear to play some causal role, but there's one kind of fat most responsible for causing type 2 diabetes: a specific type of fat stored around the internal organs in the abdomen, called visceral fat.

In most people, around 90 percent of body fat is subcutaneous fat: under the skin. When you poke your belly, the fat that feels squishy is subcutaneous. Visceral fat is not touchable from the outside, nor necessarily visible. It is sequestered behind the abdominal wall tucked in and around the organs. You can be incredibly lean and have fat around your organs. This is sometimes referred to as "thin on the outside, fat on the inside" (TOFI). Higher amounts of visceral fat do eventually reveal themselves because they expand the abdominal area, leading to a visibly larger waistline. Visceral fat is also quite hard to the touch, as it hardens the tissue that blankets the intestines. The stereotypical "beer belly" is an example of this.

Visceral fat is linked to insulin resistance and type 2 diabetes. Overweight people with diabetes have more fat in the liver and abdomen than overweight people without diabetes. In a study of more than 650,000 people in India, the presence of visceral fat increased the risk of diabetes across people classed as "normal weight," "overweight," and "obese." It was greater among those classed overweight and obese but still significant for those classed "normal weight." Another statistical analysis of a 650,000+ data set in India suggests that people in the "normal" weight category with visceral fat are more likely to develop diabetes than those who do not have visceral fat.

Why? Visceral fat releases pro-inflammatory cytokines and is more easily infiltrated by a wide variety of immune cells. This highly inflammatory process happening right there in the abdomen alongside the liver and pancreas, precious organs necessary for healthy blood sugar management, leads to insulin resistance and damage to beta cells.

As a result, people who have higher amounts of visceral fat are at greater risk of higher triglycerides, heart disease, dementia, asthma, breast cancer, colorectal cancer, prostate cancer, and type 2 diabetes. Visceral fat is associated with prolonged hospital stays, increased incidence of infections and noninfectious complications, and increased mortality in hospitals.

But not everybody has visceral fat. Some people have very high body fat percentages (lots of subcutaneous fat) but relatively low fat around the organs. Some, on the other hand, are incredibly lean, yet still have fat in their liver and other organs.

What drives the difference? Genetics, changing hormone levels, sedentary behavior, alcohol consumption, and, perhaps most important, stress.

Visceral fat has more stress hormone receptors than subcutaneous fat, and chronic activation has been suggested of the body's main stress-response system (the hypothalamic-pituitary-adrenal axis—HPA) may play a role in the development of visceral fat. Visceral fat may have a protective origin. The immune system exists to help defend us. Unfortunately, in our hugely toxified, SAD-suffused, stressful world, the system works against itself. It ends up hurting instead of healing.

Does fat loss help with type 2 and prediabetes? Usually yes, but only if you have excess fat to lose, and specifically visceral fat. When losing weight, the body will often preferentially burn fat in the liver, meaning that even just a modest amount of weight loss can help. For some people, losing just 15 percent or 10 percent of body weight can make a huge difference.

But it's important to have a broader goal than "lose weight" to fix blood sugar and heal type 2 and prediabetes. For many, it can help, but because type 2 and prediabetes are driven by damage that can come from many directions—it's most effective to supply multidimensional support. Focus on healing metabolic machinery multidimensionally.

If you think weight loss could help you, it usually happens naturally on the Yates Protocol. It happens naturally when you heal your metabolic machinery, improve insulin sensitivity, and gain healthier appetite and satiation signals so you know when to stop eating. It happens when you eat nourishing foods, eat at appropriate times, rest long and deep, incorporate exercise, strength train, and reduce stress. This is more effective than restrictive dieting focused on eating less. Bodies don't always burn fat when restricting calories, and usually the metabolic rate plummets, making it harder to lose weight in the long run and causing rebound weight gain. You can lose weight without draining your precious willpower and mental and physical energy.

Not all people need to lose weight. Not all people's type 2 and pre-diabetes includes this visceral fat. Some people have extra weight but it's all subcutaneous. Others do not have any weight to lose. It's important to assess your circumstances honestly and strategize accordingly.

Sedentary lifestyle

Sitting for long periods is a major risk factor for type 2 and prediabetes. In a review of eighteen studies including nearly 800,000 people, the greatest sedentary time compared with the lowest was associated with a 112 percent increase in diabetes risk. Sedentariness has been associated with inflammatory markers. In a recent survey of more than 127,000 adults, those who sat for six or more hours a day in their leisure time were 19 percent more likely to die in the next twenty-one years than those who spent less than three hours of leisure time sitting.

Humans are made for movement. When we keep moving, we give our bodies precious opportunities to shift out of "blood sugar storage" mode and into "blood sugar burning" mode, which helps insulin signaling pathways stay sensitive. Plus, movement keeps the muscles active as blood sugar metabolizing sites. Muscle cells use and store sugar. When in constant use, they boost metabolic rate and improve overall metabolism. Without regular movement, the wonderful blood sugar sponginess of muscles goes to waste.

Remember: Active working muscles are blood sugar sponges.

Stress

Stress puts you on a blood-sugar roller coaster, significantly damages several of the systems necessary for metabolism like the gut and the gut's microbiome, depletes the body of key nutrients, and disrupts leptin and ghrelin, leading to much more difficulty with good choices about food and health.

Stress is the most underrated cause of type 2 there is. It doesn't fit the shame and blame model, so it's easily overlooked. But it's a silent killer. It's the most common cause of type 2 diabetes because it affects everybody, though of course some more than others. In my experience, people with type 2 tend to be overtaxed: caregivers, volunteers, those working multiple jobs, doing shift work, juggling responsibilities, and who are the rocks other people always lean on.

Poor sleep

Poor sleep alone can lead to type 2. Just 1 or 2 fewer hours of sleep per night—from 7 or 8 hours to 6 hours—on average leads to a greater risk of developing type 2.

Poor sleep additionally tends to reduce resilience amidst stress by degrading brain health, blood sugar health, and all the systems necessary for supporting the body through stress.

Antibiotics and other gut microbiome killers

Antibiotics can be lifesaving, but they have a cost: They don't kill only bad bacteria. They kill good ones, too. Good bacteria help lower inflammation, support the immune system, keep blood sugar in the healthy range, break down food into important nutrients, and help the gut figure out what gets excreted and what gets absorbed into the bloodstream. Good gut bacteria help move nutrients into your bloodstream and safely keep toxins out. Without a healthy gut microbiome, both functions suffer. You don't absorb as much of the good nutrients you need, and you end up absorbing toxic by-products that wreak havoc.

A recent analysis of data from more than 800,000 women showed that a longer duration of antibiotic use in the prior four years is associated with increased risk of type 2. In a recent study of more than 200,000 people, those who took antibiotics for 90 days or more had a higher risk of diabetes. Animal models suggest antibiotics can increase insulin resistance, leading to metabolic syndrome and prediabetes.

My clinical experience confirms this. People who were put on antibiotics a lot as a kid later struggle with gut health and related diseases like diabetes. One patient, Joan, was put on repeated courses of antibiotics for ear infections as a child. This was the initial damaging event that started her on a trajectory into inflammation, insulin resistance, and type 2. If you were subjected to this kind of gut stress early on, you could end up with progressively worsening health twenty, thirty, forty years later.

Another patient, Anna, picked up a parasite while traveling and spent months enduring gut distress before being able to access proper treatment—after which her gut's microbiome had already suffered enormously. The cocktail of drugs she was put on to kill the parasite only left her microbiome more damaged.

Often, one initial blow to gut bacteria weakens the system. If not properly restored with gut-nourishing fiber and resistant starch (and probiotic foods or supplements, see the Resources on the website), the system deteriorates. The gut lining can become permeable, allowing toxins otherwise destined for excretion to pass into the bloodstream, causing the immune system to go into hyperdrive. Unaddressed, the inflammatory response grows stronger. This can cause the gut's microbiome population to become even more imbalanced, while also putting you on trajectories into developing food sensitivities, allergies, joint pain, conditions related to chronic inflammation like type 2 and prediabetes, and autoimmune diseases.

A high diversity of bacterial species protects against metabolic diseases such as obesity, prediabetes, and type 2. Lower microbial diversity increases the risk of weight gain, insulin resistance, and inflammation. An increase in pathogenic bacteria has been found in the microbiome of diabetic patients and seems to promote insulin resistance.

Healthy gut bacteria help manage those twin gremlins of appetite-signaling hormones, leptin and ghrelin. They produce a special class of molecule called short chain fatty acids (SCFA). Two short chain fatty acids, propionate and butyrate, stimulate leptin production; another, acetate, supports ghrelin secretion. These are *crucial* for healthy appetite and portion control. Emerging evidence suggests that low levels of butyrate producers increase the risk of type 2. When obese people are given an antibiotic that harms butyrate producers, they steadily develop insulin resistance. Mice treated with a butyrate precursor show protection from insulin resistance, liver disease, and obesity. Nearly everyone can benefit from intentionally supporting the gut's microbiome. But for some people, especially those with appetite difficulty, it is a dire need.

Probiotics may help. A thirty-day course of probiotics has been shown to reduce the amount of toxicity from lipopolysaccharide (LPS)—a toxic but natural part of the gut that enters the bloodstream when the gut lining has become permeable—in the blood by 42 percent. Some popularly available strains such as *Lactobacillus* and *Bifidobacterium* can improve lipid profile and reduce fasting morning blood sugars, fasting insulin, and A1C levels. Administration of *Akkermansia muciniphila* has also been proposed as an antidiabetic strategy in light of its ability to regenerate the intestinal barrier, reduce inflammation, and improve metabolic processes. Check the Resources section on the website for more information and options regarding probiotic support and supplementation.

What else helps? Fiber, complex carbohydrates, and resistant starch especially. These are excellent foods for SCFA producers and other good gut bacteria. This is why they are central in the Yates Protocol.

Healthy carbs are *healing*.

Food sensitivities

Many foods are perfectly well tolerated by a gut with tight junctures and good lubrication, that is defended by good gut microbiota. But once the gut microbiome becomes imbalanced and/or the gut lining begins to weaken, they can begin to cause symptoms like digestive issues, joint pain, and fatigue, play a role in generating or exacerbating autoimmune conditions, and contribute to the chronic inflammation and oxidative stress that drive insulin resistance and type 2.

The most common offenders are the proteins found in wheat (gluten and others), and dairy (casein and whey). These proteins are large and unwieldy. When the junctures in the intestinal walls weaken, they can begin to pass through and even further widen the junctures, leading to greater leakage of toxins and proteins that should remain in the gut into the blood. Once they pass into the bloodstream, the immune system mistakes them for toxins and flips into hyperdrive. Mice fed a gluten-free diet for forty-two weeks showed higher volumes of beta cells.

This doesn't mean that gluten and dairy proteins necessarily *cause* type 2 and prediabetes or autoimmune disease. They may in some instances, but one thing they more surely do is worsen vulnerabilities that have been created by other means. This may be why so many people benefit from removing them from their diets, whether or not they have celiac disease or other autoimmune conditions.

Having a compromised gut microbiome population can create sensitivities to almost anything. It depends on both which species are in your gut and your personal vulnerabilities. Fortunately, you can identify which foods aggravate blood sugar control and cause blood sugar to rise, with your continuous glucose monitor (CGM) or a glucometer.

Viruses

Several classes of viruses can either down-regulate the activity of beta cells or damage them. Enteroviruses, cytomegaloviruses, hepatitis C, HIV, severe acute respiratory syndrome, and COVID, among others, have been identified as triggers of both type 1 and type 2. The mechanisms of damage by viral illnesses are diverse but appear to entail liver or pancreatic injury, altered sugar and fat metabolism, and damage to mitochondria function. COVID has been shown to initiate insulin resistance and beta cell dysfunction in patients without any preexisting history of type 2 diabetes, perhaps due to a surge in production of pro-inflammatory cytokines.

Environmental toxins and our 360-degree compromise

Environmental toxins are another major cause of type 2 and prediabetes that almost no one is talking about. Talking about it would mean addressing the toxic waste products in our systems and products, and it would mean addressing disparities in public health services. Make no mistake: The role of toxins in type 2 and prediabetes is very real.

We live in a chemical soup: clothing, cosmetics, lotion, nail polish, perfumes, toiletries, diesel fumes, air and water pollution, cooking with gas, the coal used to make electricity . . . the list of contributing sources is endless.

Scientists *know* that this toxic load interferes with metabolism. It isn't conspiracy: It's fact. Environmental toxins affect the cell wall and its fluidity. They overburden the body's natural detox pathways. They impair mitochondria function, causing reduced energy and cell performance and runaway oxidative stress. They stoke chronic inflammation. All of us to some degree or another are processing this toxic load. For some this toxic burden is very great.

Air pollution is linked to type 2. Multiple studies across multiple nations have demonstrated links. A cross-sectional study of almost 3,000 adults in Iran showed that previous exposure to PM10 (particulate matter 10) for five years may be associated with higher odds of developing type 2. A study of more than 30,000 people in California showed that type 2 diabetes was associated with exposure to air pollutants like ozone, particulate matter, and nitrogen dioxide as well as proximity to traffic. Traffic police show increases in fasting blood sugars directly correlated with more time spent on traffic duty and exposed to PM2.5. In areas where there is air pollution, more vulnerable populations such as the elderly or people with low income are at greater risk, but the risk is present across various demographics and subpopulations.

Air pollution may in fact *cause* type 2. Medium-term exposure to pollutants has been associated with elevated A1C in people who didn't (yet) have type 2 diabetes, supporting the hypothesis that air pollution can play a role in the development of type 2 and prediabetes.

Mold and other microbial toxins can have similar affects as they, too, stimulate inflammation, oxidative stress, and mitochondria dysfunction. When mold grows, it releases spores and mycotoxins into the air. In mice studies, exposure to bafilomycin impairs sugar tolerance, reduces pancreatic cell function, and decreases pancreatic cell mass. Long-term exposure to ochratoxin A, a widespread toxin found in food or water-damaged houses, can cause elevated blood sugar, pancreatic damage, and lower insulin production in rats. Microcystin-LR, a toxin produced by freshwater bacteria that can be in drinking water, induces cellular stress and mitochondria dysfunction and appears to be toxic to beta cells.

One major source of toxicity we never talk about is pig feces. All over the USA, Americans consume an enormous amount of meat and poultry: on average more than 200 pounds per person per year. Concentrated animal feeding operations (CAFOs) have contracts whereby mass amounts of pigs or chickens are herded together and raised in inhumane conditions because it is cost-effective. Especially with pigs, there are large pools of excrement. The CAFOs need to get it off the property. Their awful solution: *Spray it into the air.* Whoever happens to be unfortunate enough to live around this is getting pig poop sprayed on them. These people are never the ones who are well connected politically; they're the ones without the wealth and other resources to fight back. Proximity to CAFOs has not been directly linked to type 2 and prediabetes. But I would not be surprised if it becomes an area of interest and emerges as an outcome in future studies, as proximity to CAFOs has been linked to related phenomena such as autoimmune disease, rheumatoid arthritis, anemia, cardiovascular disease mortality, and kidney disease mortality.

Research into heavy metals, industrial waste, plastic compounds, and machining fluids is ongoing. Compounds of concern include bisphenol A (BPA, a component of plastic often found in foods and drinks stored in plastic containers), diethylhexyl phthalate (another plastic by-product), perfluorooctanoic acid (PFOA, once commonly used for nonstick pans), tributyl tin (found in paint), and the heavy metals arsenic, cadmium, lead, mercury, antimony, molybdenum, and uranium. They create oxidative stress that impairs beta cell function, drives the production of inflammatory markers that hinder insulin signaling, and disrupts mitochondrial function via several pathways. They are often referred to by researchers as "environmental diabetogens."

Heavy metals polluting the water supply and agriculture may be especially damning, though few are sounding the alarms and nearly as few are listening.

The USA's Native American population is well known for having one of the highest rates of type 2 diabetes on the planet. They are almost three times more likely than non-Hispanic white adults to be diagnosed with type 2; as of 2018 they were 2.3 times more likely to die from diabetes. It is often said that these populations and other Indigenous cultures around the world are genetically predisposed to insulin resistance due to the seasonality of their diets or periods of feasting and fasting, but this is pure speculation. I suspect it's driven by racism and a refusal to take seriously the devastating effects of colonialism. Why presume there's some unsubstantiated genetic determinant driving this disparity in health outcomes when there is evidence of other causes? This narrative is an excuse to avoid facing how these communities have been and are treated.

There are causes other than toxins in the environment. One is epigenetic changes due to intergenerational trauma of being subjected to displacement, war, violence, you name it. This has epigenetic effects, as such events predispose bodies to overdetect threat (that is, to be hypervigilant), overproduce cortisol, and trigger more readily into pro-inflammatory states. Another major cause is nutrition. The US government killed off buffalo and corralled Native agriculture into poor farmland. It took all their good food away. Then the SAD steamrolled across the land. Today, many areas of Native American reservations are food deserts where cheap ultra-processed food is the most (or only) available.

Yet the greatest of all the factors may be the environmental toxins. I don't have the space here to do this complex, heartbreaking, and enraging issue justice.

For example, Navajo well water is significantly contaminated with arsenic. This well water, intended for livestock, is also drunk by humans (plus, the livestock is consumed by humans). To the best of my limited engagement with the available literature on this, as much as 30 percent of people living on Navajo lands lack access to public water systems, and up to 40 percent do not have running water. Running water may not help those who have it. Many of the public water systems on Native lands such as in Western Navajo Nation are out of compliance.

There are also more than 1,100 abandoned uranium mines and waste sites across Navajo lands. These pollute the water supply, air, and food consumed from crops grown nearby.

In one study of Native Americans living in rural and small-town communities, four forms of arsenic and uranium, as well as antimony, cadmium, lead, molybdenum, selenium, tungsten, and zinc, were detected in elevated quantities and correlated to disrupted fatty acid, energy, and amino acid metabolism pathways. Of the study participants, 50 developed diabetes within five years of the study. Arsenic and uranium were present in their samples but were not present in the samples of those who did not develop diabetes.

Are Native American and other Indigenous cultures *genetically* predisposed to type 2 diabetes? No, they're disposed because they've been and are being poisoned. I've had a chance to visit a few Native

American reservations and witness the extent—really, the lack—of public services. This is not right.

Adverse childhood experiences

Adverse childhood experiences (ACEs) are childhood traumas such as abuse, neglect, family dysfunction, and others. Events that happen early on in a child's development set the stage for how the body responds to various stimuli. One study of more than 50,000 US adults showed that childhood abuse, witnessing domestic violence, divorce, and living with someone depressed, abusing substances, or incarcerated are associated with low self-rated health, functional limitations, heart attack, and diabetes.

People who experience traumatic events in childhood appear to have a larger number of mitochondrial genomes per cell, which some researchers think develop to compensate for mitochondrial problems. This is being researched with respect to clinical psychology and psychiatric disorders, but any impairment to mitochondrial function is relevant to type 2 diabetes, especially when paired with a nervous system wired to hypervigilance and over-production of cortisol.

A review of studies on ACEs suggests a relationship between ACEs and chronic inflammation in early ages, inducing physiological changes that could be long-lasting. ACEs make the stress system hyperactive, leading to long-term stress and a hair trigger for pro-inflammatory states. ACEs are associated with a higher risk of type 2, with the odds of diabetes increasing by almost 11 percent for each additional adverse experience.

IT'S NOT YOUR FAULT

Why do you have type 2 or prediabetes? Why does anyone?

Whatever your personal causes driving your type 2 or prediabetes, they're not a lack of discipline. It's not because there's anything wrong with you. You haven't done anything wrong. There's nothing to be ashamed of. The damage has been insidious, likely coming at you from many angles, including ones that on the surface seem *healthy*, like overusing antibiotics or eating foods with "low fat" and "heart healthy" slapped on the label.

Even if you've eaten more processed food than you like, or moved less than you'd like, that's not a matter of discipline, willpower, or worth. That behavior itself is driven by how the SAD and the globalizing American way of life have been intentionally designed to maximize profits at the expense of your natural health: physical, psychological, emotional.

There are so many causes of metabolic damage: genes, intergenerational trauma, environmental toxins, early childhood traumas, viruses, antibiotics, food sensitivities, poor sleep, and stress. Type 2 and prediabetes are truly multicausal and context dependent.

Eat less, exercise more fails because even when you manage to lose weight that way, it doesn't heal the underlying damage done by the causes of type 2 and prediabetes.

WHY THE FIVE STEPS WORK

The five steps work because they heal the body's blood sugar management organs and systems.

Nutrition. Your body needs ample protein to build blood sugar management organs and systems. It needs fiber and complex carbohydrates/resistant starch to feed the gut's microbiome, which helps absorb nutrients, defends against toxic invaders, and is necessary for healthy appetite and satiation signals. It needs abundant vitamins and minerals to support insulin management systems. It needs fiber and fat to act as blood sugar sponges. A diet rich in lean protein, fiber, healthy fat, and complex carbohydrates/resistant starch is anti-inflammatory, nutrient-rich, and gut-supportive. The Yates Protocol is the ideal nutritional template.

Meal timing. Metabolism works best when in time with the natural rhythm the body was designed for. Eat in meals, don't snack, consume most of your food earlier in the day, and you empower your body to digest when it wants, burn sugar when it wants, and rest when it wants. If you intermittently fast, you amplify your blood sugar resetting abilities by giving your body a Timed Window for Healing. This means more time in a fasted state overnight to reset blood sugar, seep up remaining pathogens or other potential threats, process any buildup of toxins, and improve cognitive function and mood, among so many other things.

Sleep. When you sleep long and deep, you help your body start the next day at the lowest blood sugar level possible and with the greatest resilience to potential stressors throughout the day. Sleep is central to reducing inflammation, healing the body from oxidative stress, supporting healthy sugar and fat metabolism, and healthy ghrelin and leptin function, empowering you to eat healthy amounts of food without taxing your precious willpower.

Exercise. When you exercise, you burn through sugar and help increase insulin sensitivity. You support the blood-sugar sponginess of your muscles. You support a healthy metabolic rate. Building muscles increases your capacity to burn and store sugar. You restore metabolic fitness and flexibility, reduce inflammation, and enhance insulin sensitivity.

Stress. When you reduce and manage stress, you get off the whipsaw of the blood-sugar roller coaster. You restore the restful parasympathetic nervous system and all its benefits for health: improved digestion, improved appetite signaling, and improved mood and energy. You support healthy gut microbiome function, a more balanced immune system, and better blood sugar control.

REVERSING TYPE 2 AND PREDIABETES

You can heal your diabetic or prediabetic status. It's not curing. Cure means it will never happen again. Reversing isn't permanent, in the sense that once you get your numbers down into a healthy range you can go wild with cookies and cakes. You have a vulnerability to blood sugar dysregulation. You can restore functionality. But you will not become invulnerable. You must stay on top of your game.

Reversal is possible because your body comes equipped with the ability to manage blood sugar and keep you healthy and functioning throughout your life. But they can be knocked off kilter. It is very easy in today's fast-paced, nutrient-poor, toxified, profit-driven, blame-ridden world. You can reclaim your control and restore your health by helping your body get what it needs. Step by step, you can build healthy habits that support your metabolic machinery and keep it functioning as it should. Always do it with grace for yourself and your body. You're seizing control back from a world designed for it to be otherwise.

In this chapter you learned:

- Prediabetes and type 2 come from damage to the body's metabolic machinery, including systemic inflammation, oxidative stress, and mitochondrial dysfunction. These cause insulin resistance and damage to the beta cells in the pancreas that produce insulin.

- Sources of metabolic damage include the Standard American Diet, malnourishment, visceral fat, a sedentary lifestyle, stress, poor sleep, excessive antibiotic use and other gut-microbiome disrupters, food sensitivities, viruses, environmental toxins, and adverse childhood experiences.

- The five steps of the Yates Protocol are designed to heal metabolic machinery. Select the steps of the Yates Protocol to focus on by identifying which step(s) offer the greatest opportunities for *you* to restore balance and healing.

- "Healing" is not curing. You can reverse your prediabetes or type 2, but once vulnerable to type 2 or prediabetes, you are always vulnerable. Focus on making sustainable changes.

Conclusion

The overall message I offer is: Any difficulty you have with blood sugar is not your fault. You were born into a world of 360-degree compromise that profits off our poor health. But the power to fix it is in your hands. You can heal. Step by step, day by day, habit by habit, nourishing moment by nourishing moment.

Contrary to all the messaging that you are doomed to diabetes or poor blood-sugar health for life (and that it's your fault), your present situation is the opposite: an opportunity for healing. What amazing new feelings of health, energy, ease, control, and freedom from anxiety about health lie at your fingertips! Bodies are resilient. I am constantly amazed by how much health is restored when my patients begin implementing the Yates Protocol.

I invite you to engage the Protocol on your own terms: What's best for you? I have decades of clinical experience. I know it can help you. Diabetes is complicated, and every person's experience is different.

Start with changes that are feasible: perhaps changes like swapping out soda for unsweetened tea, adding leafy greens to breakfast, incorporating more protein, going for evening walks. These are a few relatively simple habits that have been big first wins for my patients.

If the changes you try work, great. Keep going. Add some more. If any specific changes don't seem to be super helpful, try something else.

If you find yourself off the horse, just visualize yourself getting back up on it. There's no such thing as failure, only opportunities for learning more about what works for you.

What's in store for you? My patients continually find new changes they can make to heal and improve their blood sugar control and health. They keep it up and enjoy it! The Yates Protocol is a new best friend and lifelong companion. Reversal doesn't mean cure. Reversal means restored health, and the gift of lifelong partnership with your body.

I am so excited for you on this journey. I am in your corner. Let us put the power back in your hands where it belongs and go seize it.

Meal Plans

7-DAY OMNIVORE, DAIRY-FREE, AND GLUTEN-FREE DIABETIC MEAL PLAN

Each meal remains low-glycemic, fiber-rich, and flavorful, while completely avoiding gluten and dairy.

Day 1

BREAKFAST: Scrambled eggs with spinach, mushrooms, avocado

LUNCH: Grilled salmon over mixed greens with olive oil and lemon dressing, quinoa

DINNER: Garlic-and-herb-roasted chicken thighs, black beans, mashed cauliflower, salsa

Day 2

BREAKFAST: 3-Ingredient Chia-Seed Pudding (page 222) with coconut milk, flaxseeds, raspberries

LUNCH: Turkey and avocado lettuce wraps with hummus, cherry tomatoes, olives

DINNER: Grass-fed beef stir-fry with bell peppers, broccoli, brown rice

Day 3

BREAKFAST: Smoked salmon with avocado, red onion, pinto beans, tomato slices

LUNCH: Grilled shrimp with cucumber salad (olive oil and balsamic dressing), roasted sweet potatoes

DINNER: Baked cod with lemon and dill, sautéed or roasted zucchini, quinoa

Day 4

BREAKFAST: Omelet with mushrooms, broccoli, onions, spinach

LUNCH: Chicken, roasted Brussels sprouts, avocado salad with lemon vinaigrette

DINNER: Lamb with roasted cauliflower (or Mashed Cauli-Tatoes—see recipe on page 209), hummus

Day 5

BREAKFAST: Hard-boiled eggs with turkey bacon, sautéed onions, kale, ginger, bell peppers

LUNCH: Tuna salad with olive oil and vinegar dressing, steamed sweet potatoes

DINNER: Baked salmon with asparagus, garlic-roasted chickpeas

Day 6

BREAKFAST: Gluten-Free Waffle (see recipe on page 196), chicken sausage, steamed spinach (or a handful of salad greens)

LUNCH: Grilled chicken with mixed greens, avocado, lemon vinaigrette

DINNER: Lamb chop with roasted Brussels sprouts, wild rice

Day 7

BREAKFAST: Scrambled eggs with mushrooms, spinach, kidney beans, avocado

LUNCH: Grass-fed beefburger lettuce wrap with caramelized onions, avocado, roasted sweet potato slices

DINNER: Roasted sole, sautéed snow pea greens, walnuts, steamed green beans

7-DAY PLANT-BASED, DAIRY-FREE, AND GLUTEN-FREE DIABETIC MEAL PLAN

Each meal remains low-glycemic, fiber-rich, fresh, and flavorful, while completely avoiding gluten and dairy.

Day 1

BREAKFAST: Macadamia nuts or pumpkin seeds, steamed sweet potatoes, handful of leafy green vegetables, half a banana

LUNCH: Quinoa and kale salad with lemon-tahini dressing

DINNER: Lentil and vegetable stew with cauliflower rice, olives

Day 2

BREAKFAST: Scrambled tofu with spinach, mushrooms, ginger, turmeric, half a banana

LUNCH: Chickpea and avocado lettuce wraps with mixed greens, cashews, hazelnuts, or sunflower seeds

DINNER: Stuffed bell peppers with black beans and brown rice, salsa

Day 3

BREAKFAST: 3-Ingredient Chia-Seed Pudding (see recipe on page 222) made with unsweetened almond milk, with berries, almonds or pumpkin seeds, one dried apricot

LUNCH: Mediterranean chickpea salad with cucumber, olives, lemon dressing

DINNER: Roasted squash and tempeh bowl, corn, with cashew sauce, berries

Day 4

BREAKFAST: Overnight oats with chia seeds, flaxseeds, blueberries

LUNCH: Edamame and cabbage slaw with sesame dressing

DINNER: Coconut curry with tofu and broccoli over wild rice

Day 5

BREAKFAST: Chickpea scramble with bell peppers, leeks, ginger, turmeric

LUNCH: Zucchini "noodles" with avocado pesto, cherry tomatoes, olives, orange

DINNER: Spinach lentils (dal) with quinoa, bok choy

Day 6

BREAKFAST: Three-bean salad, salsa, pine nuts or sunflower seeds

LUNCH: Roasted beet and arugula salad with walnuts and lemon dressing, a peach

DINNER: Stuffed acorn squash with pumpkin seeds, sunflower seeds, wild rice, dried cranberries

Day 7

BREAKFAST: Scrambled tofu, lentils, sautéed snow pea greens, rutabaga, apple slices

LUNCH: Buddha bowl with brown rice, chickpeas, roasted veggies

DINNER: Vegan chili with black beans and sweet potatoes

Resources

I warmly encourage you to check out the Resources section on my website: https://fixyourbloodsugar.org/resources.

I offer additional chapters, too big to fit into this book, on:

- meal planning,

- smart supplementation that kick-starts your journey with mitochondrial support and accelerates your healing with insulin sensitivity and blood-sugar management support, the underdiagnosed populations of slender type 2 diabetics and those with high and low blood sugar without diabetes,

- and *diets*: why keto, veganism, and calorie restriction seem to work sometimes but aren't sufficient answers to healing type 2 and prediabetes.

I also offer up-to-date information on CGMs, including how to access and pay for them.

The Resources section is full of even more knowledge, guidance, and programs designed to help you take these steps—no matter where you are in your journey. If you want or could benefit from any kind of support, please find me there.

Acknowledgments

Many thanks go to my patients and clients for allowing me to work with them on their health goals, including reversing type 2 diabetes and prediabetes. This book is the distillation of over thirty years of clinical work with people whose personal details encompass the breadth and depth of our common humanity.

I am in awe of the healing potential we each have that Mother Nature and God provide to support us as we access specific information and take action to make it our own so we can reclaim our health, step by step.

Thank you to my family for giving me the grace and space to create this work. I send a special shout-out to my husband, John C. Gonzalez, for his generous development and contribution of our family recipes shared here.

Thank you to Celeste Fine, Mia Vitale, Sarah Passick, and the team at Park Fine & Brower Literary Management for believing in my mission to help at least three million people reverse type 2 diabetes and prediabetes so they can live a healthy, energetic, independent life. Your outreach and advocacy are much appreciated. Thank you to

Stefani Ruper, PhD, for helping me shape this book and bring it to life. Your talent and listening skills are unmatched.

Thank you to JJ Virgin and Sam Horn for your encouragement, advice, and camaraderie at each stage of this publication journey. Your friendship and guidance are a gift.

Thank you to Lucia Watson for believing in my vision for this book and getting it to the audience it is meant to serve. Thank you to Hannah Steigmeyer and the team at the Avery imprint of Penguin Random House for your guidance through the phases of editing and publishing. Your feedback and guidance are game changers.

Notes

1. Nutrition

15 **Americans consume more than 15 times:** Simopoulos, A. P. 2002. "The Importance of the Ratio of Omega-6/Omega-3 Essential Fatty Acids." *Biomedicine & Pharmacotherapy* 56 (8): 365–79. https://doi.org/10.1016/s0753-3322(02)00253-6.

2. Meal Timing

48 **have been shown to improve:** BaHammam, Ahmed S., and Abdulrouf Pirzada. 2023. "Timing Matters: The Interplay Between Early Mealtime, Circadian Rhythms, Gene Expression, Circadian Hormones, and Metabolism—A Narrative Review." *Clocks & Sleep* 5 (3): 507–35. https://doi.org/10.3390/clockssleep5030034.

64 **fasting mimicking diet (FMD):** van den Burg, E. L., M. P. Schoonakker, P. G. van Peet, et al. 2024. "Integration of a Fasting-Mimicking Diet Programme in Primary Care for Type 2 Diabetes Reduces the Need for Medication and Improves Glycaemic Control: A 12-Month Randomised Controlled Trial." *Diabetologia* 67(7): 1245–59. doi: 10.1007/s00125-024-06137-0. Epub 2024 Mar 28. PMID: 38546821; PMCID: PMC11153305.

3. Sleep

69 **Chronic sleep deprivation, even as few:** Eckel, Robert H., Christopher M. Depner, Leigh Perreault, et al. 2015. "Morning Circadian Misalignment During Short Sleep Duration Impacts Insulin Sensitivity." *Current Biology* 25 (22): 3004–10. https://doi.org/10.1016/j.cub.2015.10.011.

69 **In a 2023 study:** Nôga, Diana Aline, Elisa de Mello e Souza Meth, André Pekkola Pacheco, et al. 2024. "Habitual Short Sleep Duration, Diet, and Development of Type 2 Diabetes in Adults." *JAMA Network Open* 7 (3): e241147. https://doi.org/10.1001/jamanetworkopen.2024.1147.

70 **20 percent of Americans get:** Fioroni, Sarah, and Dan Foy. 2024. "Americans Sleeping Less, More Stressed." *Gallup*, April 15, 2024. https://news.gallup.com/poll/642704/americans-sleeping-less-stressed.aspx.

71 **In a recent Gallup poll:** Fioroni and Foy. 2024. "Americans Sleeping Less."

73 **One study suggests that night owls:** Kianersi, Sina, Yue Liu, Marta Guasch-Ferré, et al. 2023. "Chronotype, Unhealthy Lifestyle, and Diabetes Risk in Middle-Aged U.S. Women." *Annals of Internal Medicine* 176 (10): 1330–39. https://doi.org/10.7326/M23-0728.

76 **Even for blind people:** Daniel, Ari. 2022. "Perceiving Without Seeing: How Light Resets Your Internal Clock." NPR Health Shots, "Finding Time." December 17, 2022. https://www.npr.org/sections/health-shots/2022/12/17/1139780998/light-brain-circadian-rhythms-blind.

77 **One study found:** Nagare, Rohan, May Woo, Piers MacNaughton, Barbara Plitnick, Brandon Tinianov, and Mariana Figueiro. 2021. "Access to Daylight at Home Improves Circadian Alignment, Sleep, and Mental Health in Healthy Adults: A Crossover Study." *International Journal of Environmental Research and Public Health* 18 (19): 9980. https://doi.org/10.3390/ijerph18199980.

81 **For the first time ever:** Fioroni and Foy. 2024. "Americans Sleeping Less." https://news.gallup.com/poll/642704/americans-sleeping-less-stressed.aspx.

82 **In 2023, 53 percent of women:** Fioroni and Foy. 2024. "Americans Sleeping Less."

94 **In one study of male volunteers:** Wefers, Jakob, Dirk van Moorsel, Jan Hansen, et al. 2018. "Circadian Misalignment Induces Fatty Acid Metabolism Gene Profiles and Compromises Insulin Sensitivity in Human Skeletal Muscle." *Proceedings of the National Academy of Sciences* 115 (30): 7789–94. https://doi.org/10.1073/pnas.1722295115.

95 **affects more than half:** Muraki, Isao, Hiroo Wada, and Takeshi Tanigawa. 2018. "Sleep Apnea and Type 2 Diabetes." *Journal of Diabetes Investigation* 9 (5): 991–97. https://doi.org/10.1111/jdi.12823.

4. Exercise & Strength Training

101 **by 40 percent:** Ross, Robert. 2003. "Does Exercise Without Weight Loss Improve Insulin Sensitivity?" *Diabetes Care* 26 (3): 944–45. https://doi.org/10.2337/diacare.26.3.944.

103 **A recent review:** Gaesser, Glenn A., and Siddhartha S. Angadi. 2021. "Obesity Treatment: Weight Loss Versus Increasing Fitness and Physical Activity for Reducing Health Risks." *iScience* 24 (10): 102995. https://doi.org/10.1016/j.isci.2021.102995.

109 **many rate HIIT:** Thum, Jacob S., Gregory Parsons, Taylor Whittle, and Todd A. Astorino. 2017. "High-Intensity Interval Training Elicits Higher Enjoyment Than Moderate Intensity Continuous Exercise." *PLoS ONE* 12 (1): e0166299. https://doi.org/10.1371/journal.pone.0166299.

109 **HIIT may also be more effective:** Maillard, F., S. Rousset, B. Pereira, et al. 2016. "High-Intensity Interval Training Reduces Abdominal Fat Mass in Postmenopausal Women with Type 2 Diabetes." *Diabetes & Metabolism* 42 (6): 433–41. https://doi.org/10.1016/j.diabet.2016.07.031.

109 **been shown to improve depression:** Korman, Nicole, Michael Armour, Justin Chapman, et al. 2020. "High Intensity Interval Training (HIIT) for People with Severe Mental Illness: A Systematic Review & Meta-Analysis of Intervention Studies–

Considering Diverse Approaches for Mental and Physical Recovery." *Psychiatry Research* 284 (February): 112601. https://doi.org/10.1016/j.psychres.2019.112601.

111 **sedentary jobs have increased:** Donnelly Michos, Erin. 2021. "Sitting Disease: How a Sedentary Lifestyle Affects Heart Health." Johns Hopkins Medicine. August 8. https://www.hopkinsmedicine.org/health/wellness-and-prevention/sitting-disease-how-a-sedentary-lifestyle-affects-heart-health.

111 **including type 2 diabetes, heart disease:** Farrahi, Vahid, Mehrdad Rostami, Dot Dumuid, et al. 2022. "Joint Profiles of Sedentary Time and Physical Activity in Adults and Their Associations with Cardiometabolic Health." *Medicine & Science in Sports & Exercise* 54 (12): 2118. https://doi.org/10.1249/MSS.0000000000003008.

111 **and cancer. Ideally,:** Ihira, Hikaru, Norie Sawada, Taiki Yamaji, et al. 2020. "Occupational Sitting Time and Subsequent Risk of Cancer: The Japan Public Health Center-based Prospective Study." *Cancer Science* 111 (3): 974–84. https://doi.org/10.1111/cas.14304.

113 **American adults over seventy-five:** Leppert, Rebecca, and Katherine Schaeffer. 2023. "8 Facts About Americans with Disabilities." Pew Research Center. July 24. https://www.pewresearch.org/short-reads/2023/07/24/8-facts-about-americans-with-disabilities/.

114 **One study of more than 35,000:** Shiroma, Eric J., Nancy R. Cook, JoAnn E. Manson, et al. 2017. "Strength Training and the Risk of Type 2 Diabetes and Cardiovascular Disease." *Medicine & Science in Sports & Exercise* 49 (1): 40–46. https://doi.org/10.1249/MSS.0000000000001063.

115 **Half of all women over fifty:** UC San Diego Health. n.d. "Osteoporosis Risk Factors." Accessed September 8, 2024. https://health.ucsd.edu/care/endocrinology-diabetes/osteoporosis/risk-factors/.

5. Stress

130 **can lead to serotonin depletion:** Eby, George A., Karen L. Eby, and Harald Murk. 2011. "Magnesium and Major Depression." In *Magnesium in the Central Nervous System*, edited by Robert Vink and Mihai Nechifor. University of Adelaide (Australia) Press. http://www.ncbi.nlm.nih.gov/books/NBK507265/.

130 **damage neurons, progressing:** Eby, George A., and Karen L. Eby. 2006. "Rapid Recovery from Major Depression Using Magnesium Treatment." *Medical Hypotheses* 67 (2): 362–70. https://doi.org/10.1016/j.mehy.2006.01.047.

133 **According to the National Institute:** National Institute of Diabetes and Digestive and Kidney Diseases (NIDDK). n.d. "Symptoms & Causes of Diabetes." Accessed September 8, 2024. https://www.niddk.nih.gov/health-information/diabetes/overview/symptoms-causes.

133 **One study of some 10,000 people:** Mohan, V., R. Vijayaprabha, M. Rema, et al. 1997. "Clinical Profile of Lean NIDDM in South India." *Diabetes Research and Clinical Practice* 38 (2): 101–8. https://doi.org/10.1016/S0168-8227(97)00088-0.

134 **This is highly inflammatory:** Carver-Carter, Ross. 2022. "How Stress Impacts the Microbiome and Gut Health." Atlas Biomedical. May 14, 2022. https://atlasbiomed.com/blog/how-stress-impacts-the-gut-via-the-gut-brain-axis/.

134 **been shown to impede enzymes:** Chutia, Happy, and Kyrshanlang G. Lynrah. 2015. "Association of Serum Magnesium Deficiency with Insulin Resistance in Type 2 Diabetes Mellitus." *Journal of Laboratory Physicians* 7 (2): 75–78. https://doi.org/10.4103/0974-2727.163131.

7. Testing for Success

166 **improves post-meal blood sugar numbers:** Zeevi, David, Tal Korem, Niv Zmora, et al. 2015. "Personalized Nutrition by Prediction of Glycemic Responses." *Cell* 163 (5): 1079–94. https://doi.org/10.1016/j.cell.2015.11.001.

9. Blood Sugar Science

230 **AGEs have been associated with:** Prasad, Chandan, Kathleen E. Davis, Victorine Imrhan, Shanil Juma, and Parakat Vijayagopal. 2017. "Advanced Glycation End Products and Risks for Chronic Diseases: Intervening Through Lifestyle Modification." *American Journal of Lifestyle Medicine* 13 (4): 384–404. https://doi.org/10.1177/1559827617 708991.

230 **A meta-analysis demonstrated:** Sharifi-Zahabi, Elham, Fatemeh Hajizadeh Sharafabad, Hadi Abdollahzad, Mahsa Malekahmadi, and Nadya Bahari Rad. 2021. "Circulating Advanced Glycation End Products and Their Soluble Receptors in Relation to All-Cause and Cardiovascular Mortality: A Systematic Review and Meta-Analysis of Prospective Observational Studies." *Advances in Nutrition* 12 (6): 2157–71. https://doi .org/10.1093/advances/nmab072.

230 **Approximately 1 in 3 adults:** Mayo Clinic. n.d. "Diabetic Nephropathy (Kidney Disease)—Symptoms and Causes." Accessed September 8, 2024. https://www.mayo clinic.org/diseases-conditions/diabetic-nephropathy/symptoms-causes/syc-20354556.

231 **Kidney damage is also one:** Feola, Mauro. 2021. "The Influence of Arterial Stiffness in Heart Failure: A Clinical Review." *Journal of Geriatric Cardiology* 18 (2): 135–40. https://doi.org/10.11909/j.issn.1671-5411.2021.02.004.

231 **Seventy-eight percent of people with type 2:** Thorsteinsson, Ægir. 2021. "How Many People Go Blind from Diabetes? | RetinaRisk." April 30, 2021. https://www.retinarisk .com/blog/how-many-people-go-blind-from-diabetes/.

231 **The structural changes in the eye:** Singh, Varun Parkash, Anjana Bali, Nirmal Singh, and Amteshwar Singh Jaggi. 2014. "Advanced Glycation End Products and Diabetic Complications." *Korean Journal of Physiology & Pharmacology: Official Journal of the Korean Physiological Society and the Korean Society of Pharmacology* 18 (1): 1–14. https:// doi.org/10.4196/kjpp.2014.18.1.1.

231 **Every year, 154,000 Americans:** American Diabetes Association. n.d. "Amputation Prevention Alliance." Accessed September 8, 2024. https://diabetes.org/advocacy /amputation-prevention-alliance#.

231 **so diabetic neuropathy causes symptoms:** Singh, Varun Parkash, Anjana Bali, Nirmal Singh, and Amteshwar Singh Jaggi. 2014. "Advanced Glycation End Products and Diabetic Complications." *The Korean Journal of Physiology & Pharmacology: Official Journal of the Korean Physiological Society and the Korean Society of Pharmacology* 18 (1): 1–14. https://doi.org/10.4196/kjpp.2014.18.1.1.

232 **It is present in 50 to 60 percent:** Singh, et al. 2014. "Advanced Glycation End Products." https://doi.org/10.4196/kjpp.2014.18.1.1.

232 **women are five times more likely:** Rosano, Giuseppe M. C., Cristiana Vitale, and Petar Seferovic. 2017. "Heart Failure in Patients with Diabetes Mellitus." *Cardiac Failure Review* 3 (1): 52–55. https://doi.org/10.15420/cfr.2016:20:2.

232 **presence of diabetes has been shown:** MacDonald, Michael R., Mark C. Petrie, Fumi Varyani, et al. 2008. "Impact of Diabetes on Outcomes in Patients with Low and Preserved Ejection Fraction Heart Failure: An Analysis of the Candesartan in Heart

Failure: Assessment of Reduction in Mortality and Morbidity (CHARM) Programme." *European Heart Journal* 29 (11): 1377–85. https://doi.org/10.1093/eurheartj/ehn153.

232 **AGEs are associated:** D'Cunha, Nathan M., Domenico Sergi, Melissa M. Lane, et al. 2022. "The Effects of Dietary Advanced Glycation End-Products on Neurocognitive and Mental Disorders." *Nutrients* 14 (12): 2421. https://doi.org/10.3390/nu14122421.

232 **researchers are currently exploring the link:** Akter, Kawser, Emily A. Lanza, Stephen A. Martin, Natalie Myronyuk, Melanie Rua, and Robert B. Raffa. 2011. "Diabetes Mellitus and Alzheimer's Disease: Shared Pathology and Treatment?" *British Journal of Clinical Pharmacology* 71 (3): 365–76. https://doi.org/10.1111/j.1365-2125.2010.03830.x.

232 **People with diabetes are:** Centers for Disease Control. 2024. "Diabetes and Mental Health." May 28, 2024. https://www.cdc.gov/diabetes/living-with/mental-health.html.

232 **increases the risk of depression:** Goldman, Bruce. 2021. "Insulin Resistance Doubles Risk of Major Depressive Disorder, Stanford Study Finds." Stanford Medicine News Center. September 22, 2021. http://med.stanford.edu/news/all-news/2021/09/insulin-resistance-major-depressive-disorder.html.

232 **presence of AGEs predicts/increases:** D'Cunha et al. 2022. "Effects of Dietary Advanced." https://doi.org/10.3390/nu14122421.

232 **schizophrenia and psychosis in adolescents:** Miyashita, Mitsuhiro, Syudo Yamasaki, Shuntaro Ando, et al. 2021. "Fingertip Advanced Glycation End Products and Psychotic Symptoms Among Adolescents." *npj Schizophrenia* 7 (1): 1–6. https://doi.org/10.1038/s41537-021-00167-y.

232 **higher AGE levels appear to correlate:** Eriksson, Mia D., Johan G. Eriksson, Hannu Kautiainen, et al. 2021. "Advanced Glycation End Products Measured by Skin Autofluorescence Are Associated with Melancholic Depressive Symptoms—Findings from Helsinki Birth Cohort Study." *Journal of Psychosomatic Research* 145 (June): 110488. https://doi.org/10.1016/j.jpsychores.2021.110488.

236 **but then pick up speed:** Tabák, Adam G., Markus Jokela, Tasnime N. Akbaraly, Eric J. Brunner, Mika Kivimäki, and Daniel R. Witte. 2009. "Trajectories of Glycaemia, Insulin Sensitivity, and Insulin Secretion Before Diagnosis of Type 2 Diabetes: An Analysis from the Whitehall II Study." *Lancet* 373 (9682): 2215–21. https://doi.org/10.1016/S0140-6736(09)60619-X.

236 **Insulin resistance can precede:** Tabák et al. 2009. "Trajectories of Glycaemia." https://doi.org/10.1016/S0140-6736(09)60619-X.

237 **are evident three to six years before:** Tabák et al. 2009. "Trajectories of Glycaemia." https://doi.org/10.1016/S0140-6736(09)60619-X.

237 **Currently, 1 in 3 American adults:** Mount Sinai. n.d. "Diabetes and Kidney Disease Information." Mount Sinai Health System. Accessed September 8, 2024. https://www.mountsinai.org/health-library/diseases-conditions/diabetes-and-kidney-disease.

237 **Most people with prediabetes:** Centers for Disease Control. 2024. "About Prediabetes and Type 2 Diabetes." National Diabetes Prevention Program. May 21, 2024. https://www.cdc.gov/diabetes-prevention/about-prediabetes-type-2/index.html.

237 **Without intervention, 5 to 10 percent:** Tabák, Adam G., Christian Herder, Wolfgang Rathmann, Eric J. Brunner, and Mika Kivimäki. 2012. "Prediabetes: A High-Risk State for Developing Diabetes." *Lancet* 379 (9833): 2279–90. https://doi.org/10.1016/S0140-6736(12)60283-9.

238 **when first diagnosed:** Mount Sinai. n.d. "Diabetes and Kidney Disease Information."

https://www.mountsinai.org/health-library/diseases-conditions/diabetes-and-kidney
-disease.

238   **Prediabetes increases the risk:** Centers for Disease Control. 2024. "The Surprising
Truth About Prediabetes." August 6, 2024. https://www.cdc.gov/diabetes/prevention
-type-2/truth-about-prediabetes.html.

10. Causes & Reversal Science

244   **Pro-inflammatory molecules associated:** Festa, Andreas, Ralph D'Agostino Jr., George
Howard, Leena Mykkänen, Russell P. Tracy, and Steven M. Haffner. 2000. "Chronic
Subclinical Inflammation as Part of the Insulin Resistance Syndrome: The Insulin Resistance Atherosclerosis Study (IRAS)." *Circulation* 102 (1): 42–47. https://doi.org/10
.1161/01.cir.102.1.42.

244   **Certain inflammatory markers:** Tsalamandris, Sotirios, Alexios S. Antonopoulos,
Evangelos Oikonomou, et al. 2019. "The Role of Inflammation in Diabetes: Current
Concepts and Future Perspectives." *European Cardiology Review* 14 (1): 50–59. https://
doi.org/10.15420/ecr.2018.33.1.

245   **It contributes to insulin resistance:** Rudich, A., A. Tirosh, R. Potashnik, R. Hemi,
H. Kanety, and N. Bashan. 1998. "Prolonged Oxidative Stress Impairs Insulin-Induced
GLUT4 Translocation in 3T3-L1 Adipocytes." *Diabetes* 47 (10): 1562–69. https://doi
.org/10.2337/diabetes.47.10.1562.

245   **And it directly damages beta cells:** Karunakaran, Udayakumar, and Keun-Gyu Park.
2013. "A Systematic Review of Oxidative Stress and Safety of Antioxidants in Diabetes: Focus on Islets and Their Defense." *Diabetes & Metabolism* 37 (2): 106–12. https://
doi.org/10.4093/dmj.2013.37.2.106.

246   **25 percent to 80 percent:** Kreienkamp, Raymond J., Benjamin F. Voight, Anna L.
Gloyn, and Miriam S. Udler. 2023. "Genetics of Type 2 Diabetes." In *Diabetes in
America*, edited by Jean M. Lawrence, Sarah Stark Casagrande, William H. Herman,
Deborah J. Wexler, and William T. Cefalu. Bethesda (MD): National Institute of Di-
abetes and Digestive and Kidney Diseases (NIDDK). http://www.ncbi.nlm.nih.gov
/books/NBK597726/.

246   **increase chances of developing type 2:** Kreienkamp, Raymond J., Benjamin F. Voight,
Anna L. Gloyn, and Miriam S. Udler. 2023. "Genetics of Type 2 Diabetes." In *Diabetes in America*, edited by Jean M. Lawrence, Sarah Stark Casagrande, William H. Herman, Deborah J. Wexler, and William T. Cefalu. Bethesda (MD): National Institute of
Diabetes and Digestive and Kidney Diseases (NIDDK). http://www.ncbi.nlm.nih
.gov/books/NBK597726/.

248   **cataloging 50,000 food items:** Agostino, Julia. 2022. "Database Indicates U.S. Food
Supply Is 73 Percent Ultra-Processed." *Food Tank* (blog). November 30, 2022. https://
foodtank.com/news/2022/11/database-indicates-u-s-food-supply-is-73-percent-ultra
-processed/.

248   **A recent analysis of the CDC's:** NYU Press Release. 2021. "Americans Are Eating
More Ultra-Processed Foods." October 14, 2021. http://www.nyu.edu/content/nyu
/en/about/news-publications/news/2021/october/ultra-processed-foods.

248   **Adults sixty and over:** NYU Press Release. 2021. "Americans Are Eating More." http://
www.nyu.edu/content/nyu/en/about/news-publications/news/2021/october/ultra
-processed-foods.

250   **Chronic intake of excess calories:** Boden, Guenther, Carol Homko, Carlos A. Barrero,

et al. 2015. "Excessive Caloric Intake Acutely Causes Oxidative Stress, GLUT4 Carbonylation, and Insulin Resistance in Healthy Men." *Science Translational Medicine* 7 (304). https://doi.org/10.1126/scitranslmed.aac4765.

251   **For example, when Australian Aborigines:** O'Dea, Kerin. 1991. "Cardiovascular Disease Risk Factors in Australian Aborigines." *Clinical and Experimental Pharmacology and Physiology* 18 (2): 85–88. https://doi.org/10.1111/j.1440-1681.1991.tb01412.x.

251   **In such regions, type 2:** Rajamanickam, Anuradha, Saravanan Munisankar, Chandra Kumar Dolla, Kannan Thiruvengadam, and Subash Babu. 2020. "Impact of Malnutrition on Systemic Immune and Metabolic Profiles in Type 2 Diabetes." *BMC Endocrine Disorders* 20 (1): 168. https://doi.org/10.1186/s12902-020-00649-7.

252   **Johns Hopkins Medicine defines:** Johns Hopkins Medicine. 2024. "Malnutrition." June 19, 2024. https://www.hopkinsmedicine.org/health/conditions-and-diseases /malnutrition.

252   **type 2 diabetes associated with malnutrition:** Ahmed, Ibrar, Hoor Maab Kaifi, Hira Tahir, and Adan Javed. 2023. "Malnutrition Among Patients with Type-2 Diabetes Mellitus." *Pakistan Journal of Medical Sciences* 39 (1): 64–69. https://doi.org/10.12669 /pjms.39.1.5485.

253   **Overweight people with diabetes:** Yang, Minglan, Jie Chen, Jiang Yue, et al. 2023. "Liver Fat Is Superior to Visceral and Pancreatic Fat as a Risk Biomarker of Impaired Glucose Regulation in Overweight/Obese Subjects." *Diabetes, Obesity and Metabolism* 25 (3): 716–25. https://doi.org/10.1111/dom.14918.

253   **650,000 people in India:** Gupta, Rajat Das, Rohan Jay Kothadia, and Ateeb Ahmad Parray. 2023. "Association Between Abdominal Obesity and Diabetes in India: Findings from a Nationally Representative Study." *Diabetes Epidemiology and Management* 12 (October). https://doi.org/10.1016/j.deman.2023.100155.

253   **Another statistical analysis:** Teufel, Felix, Jacqueline A. Seiglie, Pascal Geldsetzer, et al. 2021. "Body-Mass Index and Diabetes Risk in 57 Low-Income and Middle-Income Countries: A Cross-Sectional Study of Nationally Representative, Individual-Level Data in 685 616 Adults." *Lancet* 398 (10296): 238–48. https://doi.org/10.1016 /S0140-6736(21)00844-8.

253   **suggests that people in the "normal" weight category with visceral fat:** Gupta, Rajat Das, Rohan Jay Kothadia, and Ateeb Ahmad Parray. 2023. "Association Between Abdominal Obesity and Diabetes in India: Findings from a Nationally Representative Study." *Diabetes Epidemiology and Management* 12 (October-December). https://doi. org/10.1016/j.deman.2023.100155.

253   **Visceral fat releases pro-inflammatory:** Nicholas, Dequina A., Jacques C. Mbongue, Darysbel Garcia-Pérez, et al. 2024. "Exploring the Interplay Between Fatty Acids, Inflammation, and Type 2 Diabetes." *Immuno* 4 (1): 91–107. https://doi.org/10.3390/ immuno4010006.

253   **people who have higher amounts:** Shuster, A., M. Patlas, J. H. Pinthus, and M. Mourtzakis. 2012. "The Clinical Importance of Visceral Adiposity: A Critical Review of Methods for Visceral Adipose Tissue Analysis." *British Journal of Radiology* 85 (1009): 1–10. https://doi.org/10.1259/bjr/38447238.

253   **Visceral fat is associated with:** Shuster et al. 2012. "Clinical Importance of Visceral Adiposity." https://doi.org/10.1259/bjr/38447238.

254   **the difference? Genetics:** Agrawal, Saaket, Minxian Wang, Marcus D. R. Klarqvist, et al. 2022. "Inherited Basis of Visceral, Abdominal Subcutaneous and Gluteofemoral

Fat Depots." *Nature Communications* 13, article no. 3771. https://doi.org/10.1038 /s41467-022-30931-2.

254 **levels, sedentary behavior:** Whitaker, Kara M., Mark A. Pereira, David R. Jacobs, Stephen Sidney, and Andrew O. Odegaard. 2017. "Sedentary Behavior, Physical Activity, and Abdominal Adipose Tissue Deposition." *Medicine and Science in Sports and Exercise* 49 (3): 450–58. https://doi.org/10.1249/MSS.0000000000001112.

254 **alcohol consumption, and:** Sumi, Masaki, Takashi Hisamatsu, Akira Fujiyoshi, et al. 2019. "Association of Alcohol Consumption with Fat Deposition in a Community-Based Sample of Japanese Men: The Shiga Epidemiological Study of Subclinical Atherosclerosis (SESSA)." *Journal of Epidemiology* 29 (6): 205–12. https://doi.org/10.2188 /jea.JE20170191.

254 **more stress hormone receptors:** Drapeau, V., F. Therrien, D. Richard, and A. Tremblay. 2003. "Is Visceral Obesity a Physiological Adaptation to Stress?" *Panminerva Medica* 45 (3): 189–95. https://www.minervamedica.it/en/journals/panminerva-medica /article.php?cod=R41Y2003N03A0189.

255 **increase in diabetes risk:** Wilmot, E. G., C. L. Edwardson, F. A. Achana, et al. 2012. "Sedentary Time in Adults and the Association with Diabetes, Cardiovascular Disease and Death: Systematic Review and Meta-Analysis." *Diabetologia* 55 (11): 2895–2905. https://doi.org/10.1007/s00125-012-2677-z.

255 **Sedentariness has been associated:** Healy, Genevieve N., Charles E. Matthews, David W. Dunstan, Elisabeth A. H. Winkler, and Neville Owen. 2011. "Sedentary Time and Cardio-Metabolic Biomarkers in US Adults: NHANES 2003–06." *European Heart Journal* 32 (5): 590–97. https://doi.org/10.1093/eurheartj/ehq451.

255 **survey of more than 127,000 adults:** Patel, Alpa V., Maret L. Maliniak, Erika Rees-Punia, Charles E. Matthews, and Susan M. Gapstur. 2018. "Prolonged Leisure Time Spent Sitting in Relation to Cause-Specific Mortality in a Large US Cohort." *American Journal of Epidemiology* 187 (10): 2151–58. https://doi.org/10.1093/aje/kwy125.

256 **greater risk of developing type 2:** Nôga, Diana Aline, Elisa de Mello e Souza Meth, André Pekkola Pacheco, et al. 2024. "Habitual Short Sleep Duration, Diet, and Development of Type 2 Diabetes in Adults." *JAMA Network Open* 7 (3): e241147. https://doi .org/10.1001/jamanetworkopen.2024.1147.

256 **antibiotic use in the prior four years:** Yuan, Jinqiu, Yanhong Jessika Hu, Jie Zheng, et al. 2020. "Long-Term Use of Antibiotics and Risk of Type 2 Diabetes in Women: A Prospective Cohort Study." *International Journal of Epidemiology* 49 (5): 1572–81. https://doi.org/10.1093/ije/dyaa122.

256 **study of more than 200,000 people:** Park, Sun Jae, Young Jun Park, Jooyoung Chang, et al. 2021. "Association Between Antibiotics Use and Diabetes Incidence in a Nationally Representative Retrospective Cohort Among Koreans." *Scientific Reports* 11 (1): 21681. https://doi.org/10.1038/s41598-021-01125-5.

256 **Animal models suggest:** Membrez, Mathieu, Florence Blancher, Muriel Jaquet, et al. 2008. "Gut Microbiota Modulation with Norfloxacin and Ampicillin Enhances Glucose Tolerance in Mice." *FASEB Journal* 22 (7): 2416–26. https://doi.org/10.1096/fj .07-102723.

257 **Lower microbial diversity:** Crudele, Lucilla, Raffaella Maria Gadaleta, Marica Cariello, and Antonio Moschetta. 2023. "Gut Microbiota in the Pathogenesis and Therapeutic Approaches of Diabetes." *eBioMedicine* 97 (November). https://doi.org/10.1016/j .ebiom.2023.104821.

257 **An increase in pathogenic bacteria:** Pedersen, Helle Krogh, Valborg Gudmundsdottir, Henrik Bjørn Nielsen, et al. 2016. "Human Gut Microbes Impact Host Serum Metabolome and Insulin Sensitivity." *Nature* 535 (7612): 376–81. https://doi.org/10.1038/nature18646.

257 **Two short chain fatty acids:** Crudele et al. 2023. "Gut Microbiota." https://doi.org/10.1016/j.ebiom.2023.104821.

258 **Emerging evidence suggests:** Karlsson, Fredrik H., Valentina Tremaroli, Intawat Nookaew, et al. 2013. "Gut Metagenome in European Women with Normal, Impaired and Diabetic Glucose Control." *Nature* 498 (7452): 99–103. https://doi.org/10.1038/nature12198.

258 **they steadily develop insulin resistance:** Vrieze, Anne, Carolien Out, Susana Fuentes, et al. 2014. "Impact of Oral Vancomycin on Gut Microbiota, Bile Acid Metabolism, and Insulin Sensitivity." *Journal of Hepatology* 60 (4): 824–31. https://doi.org/10.1016/j.jhep.2013.11.034.

258 **Mice treated with a butyrate precursor:** Vinolo, Marco Aurélio Ramirez, Hosana G. Rodrigues, William T. Festuccia, et al. 2012. "Tributyrin Attenuates Obesity-Associated Inflammation and Insulin Resistance in High-Fat-Fed Mice." *American Journal of Physiology, Endocrinology and Metabolism* 303 (2): E272–82. https://doi.org/10.1152/ajpendo.00053.2012.

258 **A thirty-day course of probiotics:** McFarlin, Brian K., Andrea L. Henning, Erin M. Bowman, Melody A. Gary, and Kimberly M. Carbajal. 2017. "Oral Spore-Based Probiotic Supplementation Was Associated with Reduced Incidence of Post-Prandial Dietary Endotoxin, Triglycerides, and Disease Risk Biomarkers." *World Journal of Gastrointestinal Pathophysiology* 8 (3): 117–26. https://doi.org/10.4291/wjgp.v8.i3.117.

258 **Some popularly available strains:** Salgaço, Mateus Kawata, Liliane Garcia Segura Oliveira, Giselle Nobre Costa, Fernanda Bianchi, and Katia Sivieri. 2019. "Relationship Between Gut Microbiota, Probiotics, and Type 2 Diabetes Mellitus." *Applied Microbiology and Biotechnology* 103 (23–24): 9229–38. https://doi.org/10.1007/s00253-019-10156-y.

258 **Administration of *Akkermansia muciniphila*:** Cani, Patrice D., and Willem M. de Vos. 2017. "Next-Generation Beneficial Microbes: The Case of *Akkermansia Muciniphila*." *Frontiers in Microbiology* 8: 1765. https://doi.org/10.3389/fmicb.2017.01765.

259 **Mice fed a gluten-free diet:** Haupt-Jorgensen, Martin, Karsten Buschard, Axel K. Hansen, Knud Josefsen, and Julie Christine Antvorskov. 2016. "Gluten-Free Diet Increases Beta-Cell Volume and Improves Glucose Tolerance in an Animal Model of Type 2 Diabetes." *Diabetes/Metabolism Research and Reviews* 32 (7): 675–84. https://doi.org/10.1002/dmrr.2802.

259 **triggers of both type 1 and type 2:** Rajsfus, Bia Francis, Ronaldo Mohana-Borges, and Diego Allonso. 2023. "Diabetogenic Viruses: Linking Viruses to Diabetes Mellitus." *Heliyon* 9 (4): e15021. https://doi.org/10.1016/j.heliyon.2023.e15021.

259 **damage by viral illnesses:** Rajsfus et al. 2023. "Diabetogenic Viruses." https://doi.org/10.1016/j.heliyon.2023.e15021.

260 **COVID has been shown:** Montefusco, Laura, Moufida Ben Nasr, Francesca D'Addio, et al. 2021. "Acute and Long-Term Disruption of Glycometabolic Control after SARS-CoV-2 Infection." *Nature Metabolism* 3 (6): 774–85. https://doi.org/10.1038/s42255-021-00407-6.

260 **study of almost 3,000 adults in Iran:** Hassanvand, Mohammad Sadegh, Kazem

Naddafi, Mojtaba Malek, et al. 2018. "Effect of Long-Term Exposure to Ambient Particulate Matter on Prevalence of Type 2 Diabetes and Hypertension in Iranian Adults: An Ecologic Study." *Environmental Science and Pollution Research International* 25 (2): 1713–18. https://doi.org/10.1007/s11356-017-0561-6.

260 **A study of more than 30,000 people:** Meng, Ying-Ying, Yu Yu, Susan H. Babey, and Jason Su. 2023. "Long-Term Air Pollution Exposures on Type 2 Diabetes Prevalence and Medication Use." *Hygiene and Environmental Health Advances* 7 (September). https://doi.org/10.1016/j.heha.2023.100062.

260 **Traffic police show increases:** Tan, Chaochao, Yupeng Wang, Mingyue Lin, et al. 2018. "Long-Term High Air Pollution Exposure Induced Metabolic Adaptations in Traffic Policemen." *Environmental Toxicology and Pharmacology* 58 (March): 156–62. https://doi.org/10.1016/j.etap.2018.01.002.

261 **but the risk is present:** Meng et al. 2023. "Long-Term Air Pollution Exposures." https://doi.org/10.1016/j.heha.2023.100062.

261 **Medium-term exposure to pollutants:** Lucht, Sarah, Frauke Hennig, Susanne Moebus, et al. 2019. "Air Pollution and Diabetes-Related Biomarkers in Non-Diabetic Adults: A Pathway to Impaired Glucose Metabolism?" *Environment International* 124 (March): 370–92. https://doi.org/10.1016/j.envint.2019.01.005.

261 **In mice studies, exposure to bafilomycin:** Myers, M. A., K. D. Hettiarachchi, J. P. Ludeman, A. J. Wilson, C. R. Wilson, and P. Z. Zimmet. 2003. "Dietary Microbial Toxins and Type 1 Diabetes." *Annals of the New York Academy of Sciences* 1005 (1): 418–22. https://doi.org/10.1196/annals.1288.071.

261 **Long-term exposure to ochratoxin A:** Mor, Firdevs, Omur Sengul, Senay Topsakal, Mehmet Akif Kilic, and Ozlem Ozmen. 2017. "Diabetogenic Effects of Ochratoxin A in Female Rats." *Toxins* 9 (4): 144. https://doi.org/10.3390/toxins9040144.

261 **Microcystin-LR, a toxin:** Zhao, Yanyan, Qing Cao, Yaojia He, Qingju Xue, Liqiang Xie, and Yunjun Yan. 2017. "Impairment of Endoplasmic Reticulum Is Involved in β-Cell Dysfunction Induced by Microcystin-LR." *Environmental Pollution* 223 (April): 587–94. https://doi.org/10.1016/j.envpol.2017.01.061.

261 **200 pounds per person per year:** United States Department of Agriculture. n.d. "Per Capita Red Meat and Poultry Consumption Expected to Decrease Modestly in 2022." USDA Economic Research Service. Accessed September 8, 2024. http://www.ers.usda.gov/data-products/chart-gallery/gallery/chart-detail/?chartId=103767.

261 **proximity to CAFOs has been linked:** Ayala-Ramirez, Montserrat, Nathaniel MacNell, Lucy E. McNamee, et al. 2023. "Association of Distance to Swine Concentrated Animal Feeding Operations with Immune-Mediated Diseases: An Exploratory Gene-Environment Study." *Environment International* 171 (January):107687. https://doi.org/10.1016/j.envint.2022.107687.

262 **anemia, cardiovascular disease:** Son, Ji-Young, Marie Lynn Miranda, and Michelle L. Bell. 2021. "Exposure to Concentrated Animal Feeding Operations (CAFOs) and Risk of Mortality in North Carolina, USA." *Science of the Total Environment* 799 (August): 149407. https://doi.org/10.1016/j.scitotenv.2021.149407.

262 **Compounds of concern include:** Bonini, Marcelo G., and Robert M. Sargis. 2018. "Environmental Toxicant Exposures and Type 2 Diabetes Mellitus: Two Interrelated Public Health Problems on the Rise." *Current Opinion in Toxicology* 7 (February): 52–59. https://doi.org/10.1016/j.cotox.2017.09.003.

262 **and the heavy metals:** Sanchez, Tiffany R., Xin Hu, Jinying Zhao, et al. 2021. "An

Atlas of Metallome and Metabolome Interactions and Associations with Incident Diabetes in the Strong Heart Family Study." *Environment International* 157 (December): 106810. https://doi.org/10.1016/j.envint.2021.106810.

262 **They create oxidative stress:** Bonini and Sargis. 2018. "Environmental Toxicant Exposures." https://doi.org/10.1016/j.cotox.2017.09.003.

262 **"environmental diabetogens":** Bonini and Sargis. 2018. "Environmental Toxicant Exposures." https://doi.org/10.1016/j.cotox.2017.09.003.

262 **almost three times more likely:** Office of Minority Health. n.d. "Diabetes and American Indians/Alaska Natives." United States Department of Health and Human Services. Accessed September 8, 2024. https://minorityhealth.hhs.gov/diabetes-and -american-indiansalaska-natives.

262 **2.3 times more likely to die:** Office of Minority Health. n.d. "Diabetes and American Indians/Alaska Natives." https://minorityhealth.hhs.gov/diabetes-and-american -indiansalaska-natives.

263 **SAD steamrolled across the land:** McCoy, Martha. 2012. "The Rise of Obesity and Diabetes with the Adoption of a Western Diet: A Case Study of Native American Communities." *Digital Access to Scholarship at Harvard.* https://dash.harvard.edu /bitstream/handle/1/11940214/mccoy_2012.pdf?sequence=1.

263 **areas of Native American reservations:** Food Research & Action Center. 2021. "Hunger, Poverty, and Health Disparities During COVID-19 and the Federal Nutrition Programs' Role in Equitable Recovery." https://frac.org/wp-content/uploads/COVID ResearchReport-2021.pdf.

263 **are food deserts:** Move For Hunger. n.d. "How Hunger Affects Native American Communities." Accessed September 8, 2024. https://moveforhunger.org/native-americans -food-insecure.

263 **as in Western Navajo Nation:** Credo, Jonathan, Jaclyn Torkelson, Tommy Rock, and Jani C. Ingram. 2019. "Quantification of Elemental Contaminants in Unregulated Water Across Western Navajo Nation." *International Journal of Environmental Research and Public Health* 16 (15): 2727. https://doi.org/10.3390/ijerph16152727.

263 **are out of compliance:** Saffron, Jesse. n.d. "COVID-19 Shines Light on Navajo Water Contamination (Environmental Factor, June 2020)." National Institute of Environmental Health Sciences. Accessed September 8, 2024. https://factor.niehs.nih .gov/2020/6/feature/1-feature-navajo-contamination.

263 **1,100 abandoned uranium mines:** Hund, Lauren, Edward J. Bedrick, Curtis Miller, et al. 2015. "A Bayesian Framework for Estimating Disease Risk Due to Exposure to Uranium Mine and Mill Waste on the Navajo Nation." *Journal of the Royal Statistical Society: Series A (Statistics in Society)* 178 (4): 1069–91. https://doi.org/10.1111/rssa .12099.

263 **50 developed diabetes:** Weaver, Janell. 2021. "Arsenic, Uranium Mix May Increase Diabetes Risk in American Indians." National Institute of Environmental Health Sciences | Environmental Factor. November 2021. https://factor.niehs.nih.gov/2021/11 /papers/toxic-metals.

263 **Arsenic and uranium were present:** Sanchez et al. 2021. "An Atlas of Metallome and Metabolome Interactions." https://doi.org/10.1016/j.envint.2021.106810.

264 **more than 50,000 US adults:** Monnat, Shannon M., and Raeven Faye Chandler. 2015. "Long Term Physical Health Consequences of Adverse Childhood Experiences." *Sociological Quarterly* 56 (4): 723–52. https://doi.org/10.1111/tsq.12107.

264 **This is being researched:** Kwon, Diana, and *Knowable Magazine*. 2021. "Could Mito-chondria Be the Key to a Healthy Brain?" *Scientific American*, June 18, 2021. https://www.scientificamerican.com/article/could-mitochondria-be-the-key-to-a-healthy-brain/.

264 **A review of studies on ACEs:** Soares, Sara, Vânia Rocha, Michelle Kelly-Irving, Silvia Stringhini, and Sílvia Fraga. 2021. "Adverse Childhood Events and Health Biomark-ers: A Systematic Review." *Frontiers in Public Health* 9: 649825. https://doi.org/10.3389/fpubh.2021.649825.

264 **leading to long-term stress:** Kalmakis, Karen A., Jerrold S. Meyer, Lisa Chiodo, and Katherine Leung. 2015. "Adverse Childhood Experiences and Chronic Hypothalamic-Pituitary-Adrenal Activity." *Stress* 18 (4): 446–50. https://doi.org/10.3109/10253890.2015.1023791.

264 **ACEs are associated with:** Soares et al. 2021. "Adverse Childhood Events." https://doi.org/10.3389/fpubh.2021.649825.

Index